Creative Ways to Explore Identity

of related interest

Intersectionality in the Arts Psychotherapies
Edited by Jessica Collier and Corrina Eastwood
Foreword by Savneet K. Talwar
ISBN 978 1 78775 434 8
eISBN 978 1 78775 435 5

Working Within Diversity
A Reflective Guide to Anti-Oppressive Practice in Counselling and Therapy
Myira Khan
ISBN 978 1 83997 098 6
eISBN 978 1 83997 099 3

Cultural Humility in Art Therapy
Applications for Practice, Research, Social Justice, Self-Care, and Pedagogy
Louvenia C. Jackson, PhD, MFT, ATR-BC
Foreword by Dr Melanie Tervalon
ISBN 978 1 78592 643 3
eISBN 978 1 78592 644 0

Art Therapy for Racial Trauma, Microaggressions and Inequality
Social Justice and Advocacy in Therapy Work
Chioma Anah
Foreword by Beth Gonzalez-Dolginko and Alan Green
ISBN 978 1 83997 833 3
eISBN 978 1 83997 834 0

Using Art Therapy with Diverse Populations
Crossing Cultures and Abilities
Edited by Paula Howie, Sangeeta Prasad and Jennie Kristel
Foreword by Mercedes B. ter Maat and Gaelynn P. Wolf Bordonaro
ISBN 978 1 84905 916 9
eISBN 978 0 85700 694 3

creative ways to explore identity

How to Work Creatively with Intersectionality within the Therapeutic Professions

Kristina Stamatiou
and Natasha D'Aguiar

Jessica Kingsley Publishers
London and Philadelphia

First published in Great Britain in 2027 by Jessica Kingsley Publishers
An imprint of John Murray Publishing Group

1

A CIP catalogue record for this title is available from the British Library and the Library of Congress

ISBN 978 1 83997 894 4
eISBN 978 1 83997 899 9

Printed and bound by CPI Group (UK) Ltd, Croydon, CR0 4YY

Jessica Kingsley Publishers' policy is to use papers that are natural, renewable and recyclable products and made from wood grown in sustainable forests. The logging and manufacturing processes are expected to conform to the environmental regulations of the country of origin.

Jessica Kingsley Publishers
Carmelite House
50 Victoria Embankment
London EC4Y 0DZ

www.jkp.com

John Murray Publishing Group
Part of Hodder & Stoughton Limited
An Hachette UK Company

The authorised representative in the EEA is Hachette Ireland,
8 Castlecourt Centre, Dublin 15, D15 XTP3, Ireland (email: info@hbgi.ie)

Dedicated to our clients and family,
for their endless teachings and support.

Contents

All pages marked with ★ can be downloaded at http://jkp.com/catalogue/book/9781839978944

Our Stories

(I am large, I contain multitudes.)

WALT WHITMAN, 'SONG OF MYSELF', 51

Identity is a complex concept. It relates to all the aspects that make up our characteristics, qualities, beliefs and life experiences. Identity can encompass individual and collective identity. It can include a sense of self and self-understanding that is largely shaped by the society in which we live, our histories and culture. We all carry the 'multitudes' that comprise our identities with us and, as art psychotherapists, learning to make sense of our identities has been a vital part of our professional and personal development.

By way of introduction, here's a glimpse into some of the aspects that comprise our identities.

Kristina Stamatiou, art psychotherapist

I am an art psychotherapy practitioner, born to immigrant parents of Cypriot heritage. I am an able-bodied, heterosexual, divorced, light-skinned woman of colour. I was born into a working-class family. I had the privilege of studying in higher education.

After the first week of my MA Art Psychotherapy course, I wanted to quit. I remember the intensity and overwhelm I felt. Looking around the lecture room, I wondered where I could place myself. Feelings of otherness consumed me. Most of the students were mature, middle-class, white women. Imposter syndrome was present and, to be honest, sometimes still is!

While I was on the programme, I noticed the gap in the recommended art therapy training literature around identity and culture. This felt incompatible with our profession. How do we begin to understand ourselves, and sensitively support our clients in doing the same, when we are not allowing space from the outset for this topic to be reflected upon and taught about?

My 'otherness' was apparent on the course, from the sound of my North London accent to my age and my appearance.

The liquid eyeliner I wore became a topic of conversation, along with how young I looked to be studying to become a therapist. I felt a sense of fetishising from my peers towards my eye makeup. Comments such as 'it must take you a long time to perfect that eyeliner' or 'you look so exotic, especially when you wear your eyeliner' were said in a way that often felt uncomfortable. However, there were no actual questions directed towards me about my choice of makeup. If people had simply asked, I could have explained.

For me, eyeliner was not solely to do with modern Western beauty standards or femininity. Instead, the tradition of wearing eyeliner was passed down to me via the women in my family. I would watch my grandmother, mother and sister apply it, looking forward to the time I got to wear it. Eyeliner is a part of my identity – a form of connection to the women in my family and to my cultural heritage. For me it is about power, womanhood and pride.

People might judge my use of eyeliner as a choice to be stereotypically feminine, an implication that I must be accepting stereotypical gender roles and rules. Whereas in fact, I was embracing my own definition of femininity, making me feel powerful and creative.

My life experiences almost felt redundant. Much of this felt like it was to do with my age. I often felt as though I needed to suppress a part of my identity to complete the course. I would avoid speaking when questions were asked, avoiding drawing attention to my accent or even to myself at all.

Today in the United Kingdom, it can cost an average of £22,000 to study an undergraduate degree and an average of £17,000 postgraduate. The only way that I was able to fund the course was to have two, sometimes three, jobs. I was working as a teaching assistant, a typist for a legal firm and a pharmacy assistant at a local supermarket. This was not the case for many of the other students on the course. People who do not have financial security to fall back on will struggle to put themselves forward. The undercurrent of classism of higher education has alienated many working-class people.

I loved going clubbing as a respite from the demands of the postgraduate course. There, I felt a sense of community that transcended race, gender and culture. However, I kept this activity secret. There was a need to adopt a 'serious' persona, not to give too much away, and to blend in with the other students. I suppose I held onto fear of being 'caught out' as not being like the rest, which in turn in my mind meant not belonging on the course, and certainly not as a trainee therapist! I was rejecting parts of my identity of which, at the time, I felt ashamed. These were the parts which did not assimilate into Western therapists' cultural identity.

However, over time, I came to value my 'otherness' as a therapist. While it made me feel separate from some of my cohort, it began to make me feel closer to my clients. I learned the value of being able to relate to my clients, to humanise myself.

Eventually, this led to me sharing layers of my identity with my peers. I offered them a choice and chance to become curious about me and my experiences. To decide to shrink myself to fulfil a certain idea of 'a therapist', due to the lack of representation within the training room, felt both unjust and counterproductive. Doing so stopped me being conscious of my own advantages and disadvantages, stunting my curiosity and my ability to be present in my working relationships.

My identity

My mother was a refugee. At age 14, she came to the UK, without her parents, fleeing the 1974 military invasion (also referred to as the Cyprus intervention), which to this day leaves the island partitioned.

My father was born in Cyprus. He moved to the England with his parents in 1960, aged two, the same year Cyprus received its independence from the United Kingdom.

The identity of Cyprus itself is long debated. Some see Cyprus as part of Europe, others, the Middle East and/or Western Asia. The history of colonisation in Cyprus dates to ancient times. The island has been ruled by the Assyrian, Egyptian, Persian, Byzantine, Roman and Ottoman Empires, among others.

The British military bases on the island remain in active use to this day. Languages spoken in Cyprus include Greek, Turkish, Cypriot Greek, Cypriot Turkish, Sanna or Cypriot Arabic, Kurbetcha (Romani Turkish) and English. The island holds its own trauma. Its capital, Nicosia, is split in two by a heavily armed border.

Due to its long history of colonisation, some Cypriots look more European, others more Middle Eastern, with different skin tones and hair texture.

From an early age, my sister and I became aware of colourism. My sister has a darker skin tone, and I am lighter skinned. We often faced contradicting messages when it came to our appearance. My sister was told to stay out of the sun because she was beginning to look 'too dark', yet I was encouraged to soak up the sun and 'get some colour'. This happened both within our Cypriot community and out of it.

After holidays, my tan was often seen as glamorous. My tan was seen as a luxury, it represented freedom, relaxation and vacation. My racial ambiguity was perceived as a benefit due to its proximity to whiteness.

Yet my sister's darker tan meant she experienced discrimination. I have been in conversations with my sister to understand her personal experience growing up as a darker-skinned Cypriot. She explained that she felt connected to her 'Cypriotness', especially when she was in Cyprus with our grandfather, who was darker skinned.

Like me, there was an ambiguity to her heritage. People would ask, 'Where are you from?' She explained that there were times she felt intimidated by this question or even fetishised, with people commenting on her 'lovely skin tone' and 'big eyes'.

There was caution when she would go out with friends, being mindful of which places were more diverse and inclusive. At times, she found that people would not hold eye contact with her or would look away as an attempt to avoid engagement. I wonder whether this was its own form of 'othering', an inability to 'see' the person – being fearful of the person that may not look like you.

Although I consider myself fortunate to have grown up in North London around other Cypriots, there was still discomfort in the air. We were often called 'bubbles'[1] and Palmers Green was referred to as 'Palmers Greek' by non-Cypriots within the area. It would be said that it was as though Palmers Green had experienced its own 'invasion' of Cypriots. Leaving aside their error in equating all Cypriots as Greek, this 'humour' from non-Cypriots was uncomfortable. Their comments subtly implied that we did not 'belong' and undercut my sense of belonging to an area I had known my whole life.

These memories of how my identity interacted with the world are ones I carry with me. As practitioners and as clients, we can grow from reflecting and explore our many layers of identity both personally and relationally.

Working in the mental health sector

In 2019, the British Association of Art Therapists survey revealed that approximately 93 per cent of UK practitioners are white (Eastwood 2021). The underrepresentation of people of colour in art therapy makes it difficult for minoritised communities to imagine themselves within the profession.

I have been on multiple job interviews in the mental health sector where the panel staring back at me all presented as white, middle-class women. The exception would be if a senior member of staff was present – they were often a white man. I became more conscious of my working-class North London accent during these interviews. I felt almost as if who I was and the job I was applying for could not align.

My own experiences around identity influenced my perspective of the helping profession and who we employ to work within organisations. In one of my professional roles, when recruiting, I noticed many of the applicants' names appeared to have been anglicised. The names on their passport would differ from the one on their covering letter, or their birth name would also appear on their CV in smaller print. I often wondered about the individual's heritage and the impact of colonialism when reading these names. I would think about colonialism and its influence, leading to the anglicisation of names over generations.

---

1 'Bubble and squeak' (usually shortened to 'bubble') has also entered the lexicon of Cockney rhyming slang as a term – usually rather derogatory – for someone of Greek heritage.

At times it felt like an impossible task to build my identity as an art psychotherapist, due to the lack of representation and diversity within the profession. This is what pulled me towards the broader arts community. Meeting artists from many backgrounds, openly discussing our similarities and differences, showed me that there were spaces in which we share common struggles and inspirations. Meaningful connections were made. Creative spaces became collective spaces. Discussion around oppressive systems and power were at the centre of discourse around mental health.

Back on the first day of the course, I heard a gentle and familiar accent coming from across the room: a Londoner. I did not know it then, but it was the voice of the person who would one day be the co-author of this book.

Our meeting that day allowed me to hold on to a sense of belonging and possibility, which helped shape my clinical practice and identity as a therapist. Drawing on our experiences together on the course, sharing our advantages and disadvantages, and our similarities and differences, provided the foundations of our friendship. We learned together that we had a voice that required us to not stay silent and that we shared the same desire for action and change within our profession.

A way in which we can all help is by challenging the status quo and working with other professionals and communities to encourage change through collective action.

We should also be able to reflect on our therapeutic work with a client, by being able to address our differences and similarities within the therapeutic space together and outside of the therapeutic space. We should be able to address our differences, our oppressions and our privileges: not only with our clients but also with our colleagues, promoting social change through our work.

We began to have conversations with the university where we trained about adapting the current MA Art Psychotherapy curriculum. We collaborated on developing new modules that would be added to the programme. The new curriculum now considers anti-discriminatory practice and intersectionality, topics on which my co-author and I have lectured.

Our endless conversations around identity and culture within therapy, whilst studying and practising, were a necessity to challenge, listen, speak and, hopefully, move towards a profession which can facilitate structural change and movement.

Natasha D'Aguiar, art psychotherapist

As a child, strangers would come up to me and my brother to comment on our appearance. They would exclaim over his blue eyes and my green ones, our blond curls and brown olive-toned skin. Fetishising us even as children.

For many, there is a sense of loneliness when you are mixed race. It feels like a unique experience. You can't share with immediate family as they are 'different' races to you. You can't share with friends as they don't have the same heritage. I felt lucky to have a brother who shared both the 'ambiguous' heritage and questions from others.

For ease, when people would ask me where I was from (often in the first sentence when they met me), I would say: 'My mum's white and my dad's black, from Guyana. Not Ghana, Guyana.' But of course, this is a simplification. When we offer these simple answers, we ignore our vast, complex heritage that we carry from generations before.

My mum is from London in England. Her mother was born in India, in what can be called British India, the British Raj, Crown rule in India or the Indian Empire, but would say she was from England. My dad is from Guyana, South America, which is part of the Caribbean.

Growing up, I disliked the attention my 'difference' brought and I felt this discomfort in my body. When people told me I had a lovely 'tan', it felt like another form of objectification. People told me to take these comments as compliments, but it did not feel that way.

In my environment, it seemed to me that most of the white girls wanted darker skin and the Black community idealised 'light skinned' girls. While I did not internalise comments about my skin tone, I internalised similar comments about my hair and eyes. I wished I was not so 'different' and wanted to blend into the crowd. Standing out in any way was something I avoided growing up.

In primary school, sitting on the carpet during reading time, other children used to play with my hair. Throughout my childhood, I had my hair played with, touched, spoken about and fetishised for being different and unusual. My hair made me 'exotic' and 'unique' but also brought a lot of unwelcome attention. By the time I was eight, I instructed my mum to cut it short. Looking back, this feels like a protest against the attention I was receiving. Thankfully, my mum encouraged me to be myself and do what I wanted with my hair.

I attended a majority-white secondary school for girls where the students and teachers would compliment my hair, but would also constantly suggest that I straighten it. 'I love your hair, why don't you change it completely' was what I heard internally. I did not know how to receive this because it felt like an insult. *They love my hair so much, but they want it to be like theirs.*

An objectifying gaze had been upon me from childhood, when I could not respond. It was common for men to beep their car horns when they drove past me in my school uniform, or to approach me in the street or at a bus stop. I could not speak up because I did not have the language.

Even though I knew I would receive comments, no matter how quiet I was, or how covered up my body was, I acted in a way to avoid drawing any extra attention to myself. When you feel as though you don't look like anyone else, attention is the enemy.

A male colleague once asked me how I was going to handle objectification by male clients. I remember thinking that I had to handle this my whole life! I could not imagine why it would be any different in a mental health setting. This felt significant for me because I realised how my outside life intersected with my professional role and how I brought my identity and experiences with me.

Becoming a therapist and integrating my identity

On my journey to becoming an art therapist, my identity again influenced my experience and my steps forward in the profession.

My art therapy training gave me so much, but I also recognise that it was developed from a Westernised approach to therapy from a mostly white, male lens. I remember wondering where my place in the therapeutic landscape would be, and where I would fit in. Now I realise that it is not about fitting in but about what we can bring that is different. How what we bring can be valued is the more pertinent question.

If I were to share my thoughts around my identity in the therapy room, how can the therapist best understand and work with these experiences? I have been driven to co-create this book as direction for therapists, and anyone working with people, to explore and unpick aspects of identity without making assumptions. To give something I would have liked to have received, to give space to this exploration with curiosity and safety.

Starting my MA felt like a familiar environment for me, in that I once again felt 'different'. Most of the spaces and educational spaces I had experienced in the past made me feel 'other'. This was the case on the MA. The course cohort was mostly white middle-class women, which is representative of the profession of art therapy. Entering this profession was not different for me, as I have been 'othered' for most of my life. It was not going to end there and it felt okay at the time. In fact, it would have felt stranger if everyone were from a similar background and heritage to my own.

Due to my educational privilege, I was able to go to university. My parents gave me the opportunity to do what I wanted to do. They instilled in me the mantra 'I can'. My parents were not necessarily able to fulfil their own hopes and dreams, but they knew that I could. They gifted me the mindset that I can achieve – that I am 'good enough'.

Although my parents and the generations before them did not go to university, I was encouraged to do so. To carry my working-class roots into a world of middle-class privilege, with colleagues who became friends, who had vastly differing experiences from me.

When I met Kristina and we formed our close friendship, and then our partnership within our art therapy world, I found community. Hearing a similar accent speaking eloquently, I knew I had found a friend with whom I could share my experience of university and the profession. Kristina would validate my experience. We would share our feelings of otherness but also acknowledge our privileges. Often, we would talk about what brought us to this point, reflecting on our histories and what we could bring to the work.

We shared many values, passions and hopes. This was a blessing in space where I was not sure how to be. I would question what I wore and how I presented myself. A clear memory was how I tried to make my style of dress plainer to 'fit in'. 'Do art therapists wear Dr Martens?' I asked myself.

I did not think so! But with Kristina, I felt more comfortable expressing myself. I realised my difference and unique identity could bring value.

Saving up for the expensive MA and taking in every drop of knowledge was an aim we shared. We were careful not to miss anything or waste the experience.

There was much talk about finding honorary contracts where you work for free, or voluntary roles, to gain experience, but Kristina and I shared that unspoken hustle that rages within the working class. We dared to find work in an environment that was hard to find employment.

The course, at that time, lacked any focus on difference. This was disappointing but reflective of the contemporary standard. During my own therapy and clinical supervision, I felt talking about identity and difference in the therapy room was a missing element. We had not been trained to explore or notice it, but as I have always been 'different', I could not ignore its presence in the therapeutic or supervisory relationship.

The murder of George Floyd by police in the USA had a significant impact on me. Before this incident and the ensuing global outcry, I felt a need to not draw attention to myself and my difference. Since his death, seeing people stand in solidarity together fighting against racism, I began to speak out about my experiences of difference, to tell my story and connect with others.

My identity and experiences were intrinsic to my practice, and I wondered how clients' identities could be best supported in the therapy room through creativity.

Kristina and I began asking the first of many questions about race, culture, age, gender and more in therapy, and we wondered why, in our experience, these conversations were not yet central. We had clinical questions we felt we could not share within our therapy circles. This book encompasses those questions for others who may be whispering the same words. Working directly on identity was something we began developing in our therapeutic practice.

Slowly, we were able to bring this into our client work. We noticed clients would rarely speak about their identity or culture, unless asked directly. Over time we thought together about ways to explore this in a creative way, drawing on our training as art therapists and bringing the rich experiences of others to our work. This is how this book came about.

Introduction

Why use creativity to explore identity?

> *...creative connection is the use of creativity to access and feel connection and get yourself and those with you in the moment into a more connected space.*
>
> KAE TEMPEST, *ON CONNECTION* (2022, P.8)

Connection is integral to our wellbeing; we all benefit from a sense of belonging and feeling understood. As art psychotherapists, we work with clients to explore their complex identities using creative approaches. Creativity, defined by the *Cambridge Dictionary* as 'the ability to produce *original* and unusual ideas, or to make something new or *imaginative*', is not an exclusive practice reserved for gifted artists, as some people might initially assume. Creativity is for everyone and extends far beyond the boundaries of painting a picture.

When we refer to creativity in this book, we refer to the *act of making*. Whether making a mark on a page, having a meaningful conversation or constructing a new idea, this is being creative. Our creativity can be channelled in different ways to support our understanding of ourselves and others. It is key to life – we see it expressed throughout our day-to-day activities, from choosing what to wear in the morning to making dinner in the evening.

Being creative in the broadest sense of the word can help us access and explore feelings in a way that talking may not. Sometimes it offers a gentle way to explore difficult topics, such as identity, and can promote connection. This book is for therapists and clinicians who are working with their clients to understand and illuminate the importance of identity.

It is also for those who want to understand how identity and creativity might intersect in the therapy room.

By introducing key theoretical constructs relating to creativity and identity in Part 1, and by sharing ideas for therapeutic creative activities in Part 2, we hope to provide a constructive framework for you to support your clients to better understand and accept themselves.

Robust research evidence supports the value of using non-verbal creative methods to support psychological recovery. In *The Body Keeps the Score* (2014), psychiatrist Bessel van der Kolk describes the reliance of mainstream Western psychology on verbal therapies in contrast to the use of movement and breath, as well as practices including rhythmic drumming, Taekwondo and Capoeira, in other regions and cultures. Moreover, he argues that 'talking isn't enough and that bodies remain hypervigilant' unless somatic methods are used (2014, p.248). While these creative and expressive alternatives are not yet always mainstream, their value is increasingly being recognised within the Western approach and within organisations such as the National Health Service (NHS), that have traditionally used talking therapies as the primary therapeutic model.

Travelling to an 'unseen world'

> *...the act of creation is an attempt to enter a mysterious realm. A longing to transcend. What we create allows us to share glimpses of an inner landscape, one that is beyond our understanding. Art is our portal to the unseen world.*
>
> RICK RUBIN, 'THE UNSEEN', *THE CREATIVE ACT: A WAY OF BEING* (2023)

Using creativity to explore identity can bring people in touch with their authentic self. Creative methods can be particularly constructive when clients have found it challenging to talk about themselves. Experimenting with creative methods may enable some clients to feel more comfortable sharing aspects of their inner world and identity; making or expressing something non-verbally can create a 'portal' to a place of enhanced understanding. Creative activities can encourage greater self-awareness by externalising aspects of a client's identity. When we collaborate with clients on the activities in this book, we are asking them to go into the realm of the 'unseen' and to activate their spiritual self.

A spirit of openness and curiosity is foundational to any therapeutic work that explores identity. As practitioners, we have experienced negative identity-based assumptions in therapy circles and we have made our own mistakes by not fully taking clients' identities into consideration. Acknowledging the importance of identity has been a blind spot in our profession for too long, but we are moving into a state of change. The desire to accelerate this change has inspired our book. We hope that it enables you, as a practitioner, to work creatively to explore identity with your clients.

How to use this book

Have you ever wanted to develop your 'non-judgemental practice' but not known how to? Blending theoretical and practical approaches, this book:

- Offers guidance that will enable you to engage in challenging therapeutic conversations about identity
- Outlines flexible creative activities to try with clients
- Proposes ideas for making therapeutic sessions more inclusive.

It can be daunting to ask someone about their experiences of difference or intersectionality (see A Note on Terminology), but if we don't ask, aren't we doing a disservice to our clients? Avoiding identity-based questions may protect us from feeling vulnerable as clinicians, but what do we lose in the process? The instinct to shy away from difficult conversations because we find them challenging to navigate is common, but mere curiosity about a client's experiences is not sufficient for fostering inclusivity and engaging in meaningful identity work.

We wrote *Creative Ways to Explore Identity* because we have learned that providing open space may not be enough to enable our clients to bring all of themselves into therapeutic sessions. This book contains tools to build your confidence in starting uncomfortable conversations with clients in a creative, holistic way. We do not claim to be experts, but we hope that our creative approaches can provide scaffolding to support people in their therapeutic journey.

We believe that therapists are drawn to the 'helping professions' by the desire to help others. However, when it comes to intersectionality, therapists are not always trained to make connections or to see the therapeutic encounter through an intersectional lens. But there is so much to be gained by learning to hold clients' identities in mind. As art psychotherapists, much of our approach is creative and interpersonal; this book will show you how creative methods can be used to reach a more holistic understanding of your clients. It intends to inspire the tentative curiosity needed to awaken identity and to uncover intersections within the world our clients inhabit. Part of this process also involves starting to recognise our own biases.

The activities in this book can be used as experiential exercises together with other professionals, but also with our clients in sessions, together or independently.

Reflect on your intentions

Before you use this book, please consider the following questions to explore your therapeutic intentions and aims:

- Why are you using this book?
- What are your aims for the therapeutic invention?
- Where does your interest in creatively exploring identity come from?

It could be useful to refer to clinical supervision or a mentor for support and advice.

Collaborate with clients

Collaboration with clients and their therapeutic goals is imperative to the working relationship, whether this be in psychotherapy, counselling or social work. Clients are the expert by experience, and this should be at the fore of your work with them. If you use a directive activity (e.g., 'Transforming inner scripts' in Chapter 7), you should seek permission from your client to ensure that they fully understand and can engage with the process. This will look different for each distinct client group (e.g., children and families, adolescents, adults, couples or older adults) and organisational setting.

Take a flexible approach to the activities

Although we provide a basic example of how each activity can be used, in therapeutic practice please adapt the activities flexibly to your client, setting or organisation. None of the activities are fixed but instead offer a fluid route towards exploring identity. Although the activities can be introduced in a directive manner, they do not need to be, and if a client organically adapts an activity as their creative process deepens, this should be embraced and supported, and it can be used as a stepping stone. Similarly, if a client wishes to focus on an activity over several weeks, this is also okay. Activities can last an hour, or across several weeks, depending on different clients' preferences, and it is also possible to adapt the activities to suit the varied needs of each developmental stage in the therapeutic process.

Pitfalls to avoid

This book is a gateway to exploring the complex and sometimes challenging subject of identity in an interesting and creative way. Used flexibly, we hope that it will support clients' personal development and healing. However, therapeutic work on identity can be demanding, and there are some common pitfalls to avoid along the way:

- *Remember that this is a tool, and not a manual or a 'how to...':* You do not need to follow the activities in sequence or prescriptively stick to the guidelines. Explore the possibilities of different activities in supervision or with peers, if this feels appropriate.

- *Do not assume that you are the expert:* There are no fixed ways of correcting someone's difficulties, and we are not about fixing human experience. The aim of the book is to use creativity to help a client better understand themselves. Everyone has unique experiences of what it is like for them to navigate the world. Keep an open mind and take a collaborative and person-centred approach.

- *Steer clear of strict agendas:* Challenge your own expectations and allow your client to respond flexibly to activities and lead the direction of therapy.

- *Limit the ambition to explore everything:* It is not possible to comprehensively explore every aspect of a client's identity, so be led by what they bring to the sessions and go at their pace.

A Note on Terminology

Several key words and terms are used throughout this book. Please read this list for clarification of what we mean in our use of these terms. Please note that although these definitions are current, language evolves, and future interpretations of these words may be different.

Colonisation When people take over and occupy Indigenous people's land, exercising control over them and their land.

Culture This may relate to someone's heritage or the systems that they are part of, for example the cultural norms within someone's family or the cultural customs within their society. It refers to the shared beliefs that categorise a group of people or society.

Ethnically minoritised people This refers to all ethnicities excluding white British. We have written this book from our perspective and experiences as women of colour in the UK. As writers, there is no term that sits entirely comfortably with us, and we recognise that the same may also be true for our readers.

Gender This does not relate to the biological sex of a human being, but to a fluid gender that may differ from the gender assigned at birth.

Identity This relates to all aspects of our characteristics, qualities, beliefs and life experiences. Identity can include individual and collective identity. It can encompass a sense of self and self-understanding that is largely shaped by the society in which we live, as well as our histories and cultures.

Intersectionality This refers to how the different elements of identity – such as gender, race, spirituality, ability and ethnicity – combine and influence each other to shape someone's experiences. An intersectional approach acknowledges that aspects of identity do not exist in isolation but are interconnected and affect how someone navigates the world. When different aspects of a person's identity interact, they can create unique vulnerabilities. For example, an immigrant with disabilities may face multiple simultaneous barriers, such as with employment and the healthcare and legal systems.

LGBTQIA+ This refers to people who are lesbian, gay, bisexual, transgender, queer, intersex or asexual plus. There is no term that can encompass the entirety of sexual and gender expression.

Service users/clients These are the members of the public you work with, for example children and young people, adults or older people.

Session We have used this term because it sits within our formalised learning construct as trained art psychotherapists. When we refer to a session, this could mean a meeting, an interaction, a therapeutic intervention or an appointment.

PART 1

Key Theoretical Constructs

CHAPTER 1

Frameworks

This chapter explores frameworks that can be used within psychotherapy and counselling. These can help to provide a structure for exploring the complex phenomena around identity and culture within a therapeutic context. However, it is important to note that they may not be universally applicable – different frameworks may be more or less useful than others, depending on our clients. As Jonathan Rose, an American historian, said: 'We can also become stuck in a frame and judge everything by it, as in the old joke about the psychoanalyst who wonders what his doorman really meant when he said "good morning"' (Rose 2021, p.8).

Intersectionality

As we start this section, it is important to note that this book's focus on intersectionality and identity politics primarily examines the contributions of activists and scholars from the West. We acknowledge the crucial work of individuals from many other backgrounds and perspectives, including Black feminists, queer disability scholars, lesbians of colour, Latinas and voices from Asia, all of whom have played a vital role in shaping and advancing the concept of intersectionality.

Two have been significant in our developing understanding of identity: Amina Mama, a Nigerian-British feminist scholar, whose work centres around post-colonial feminism and stresses the importance of understanding how intersections of identity, such as gender, race and neocolonialism, cut across in African societies, and Siti Musdah Mulia, an Islamic feminist scholar from Indonesia. Mulia's work centres on and advocates for the representation of gender equality within an Islamic framework. Her work highlights that identity and culture intersect in ways that are context-specific, looking particularly at Southeast Asia.

What is intersectionality?

Intersectionality is a framework that we use to help us understand how different aspects of a person's social and political identity, such as gender, class and race, intersect to create experiences of privilege and oppression.

During the 1980s and 1990s, institutions began responding to the social movements and activism of the 1960s and 1970s, particularly concerning exclusion within professional environments. These responses included efforts to recruit more individuals from marginalised groups into workplaces. The goal was to initiate efforts to address and mitigate systemic inequalities that had persisted for decades.

Social movements such as the Women's Liberation Movement (1960s–1980s) were accompanied by ground-breaking contributions from a group of US Black feminist activists known as the Combahee River Collective (1974–80), who brought the concept of 'identity politics' into mainstream awareness (Taylor 2017, p.4). They emphasised that oppression was shaped by multiple interlocking systems, which collectively created unique and compounded forms of suffering. This perspective underscores the need to examine oppression through diverse experiences and lenses. The Combahee River Collective recognised that Black feminists did not have the same experiences as white feminists, and that Black women would not have identical experiences of racism as Black men. They needed to create room for discussions around the Black female experience that was missing from the white feminist discourse.

Kimberlé Crenshaw, an African American professor of law and critical race studies theorist, coined the term 'intersectionality' in an article in 1989, and popularised the way in which we understand the concept. Her article explored how the traditional form of looking at discrimination through one axis fails to look at the overlapping and interconnecting forms of oppression experienced by people who belong to various marginalised groups. For example, historically, feminist and legal frameworks addressed race and gender separately; this compartmentalisation neglected the experiences of Black women who would have faced discrimination at the intersection of both gender and race.

In contrast, the intersectionality framework views forms of oppression as interconnected rather than separate and independent. A person can simultaneously fall within multiple facets of identity, where their privileges and oppressions will fluctuate. Each social group that a person is part of affords them with unmerited advantages but also disadvantages.

> **Maya is a 22-year-old Black queer woman** and a first-generation university student. Maya's parents are divorced. Her father lives in Somalia. Maya's mother is a full-time carer for Maya's sister, who has mobility issues. Alongside studying part-time, Maya works two part-time jobs to help her mother with bills and general living costs. Maya struggles with anxiety, which often affects her sleep. The intersections of Maya's race, sexuality, socioeconomic background and her responsibilities as part of a single-parent caregiving household places Maya at greater risk of systemic discrimination. These overlapping identities can lead to fewer opportunities, increased bias and exclusions. She experiences exclusions in access to financial support and resources, and exclusions in academia and professional settings. Access to these would have helped to support her in her current circumstances.

Bringing an intersectional approach into therapy

Adopting an intersectional approach within therapy involves acknowledging that everyone has multiple layers of identity. As therapists or practitioners, we are not exempt from power dynamics. We must be alert to the complications and entanglement in the relationship between a client and therapist or practitioner. Both the therapist or practitioner and client in any therapeutic relationship will have had complex, interconnected experiences of social inequalities and structures, and this should be considered within the relationship in a holistic manner. Facilitating an intersectional way of working with a client in therapy allows us to look at the world through multiple lenses. People are complex, and so is the world and environment in which they live. This way of working allows that complexity to enter the space, to build and reflect on the relational.

To illustrate how different elements of identity overlap and combine to create someone's identity, we have created our own intersectionality diagram and activity. The diagram shows a visual representation of the overlapping layers of identity. The blank diagram can be used to explore the intersections of a client's identity within a therapeutic session, and can be adapted to represent different elements and experiences of identity.

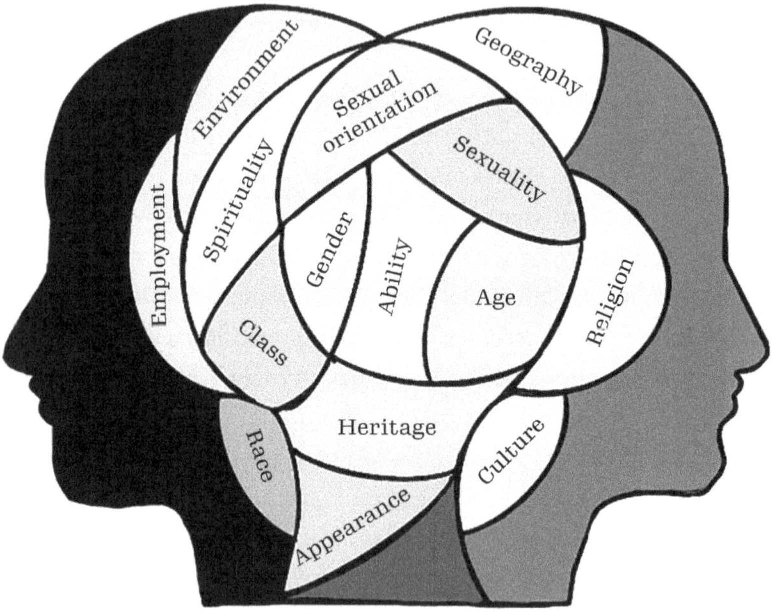

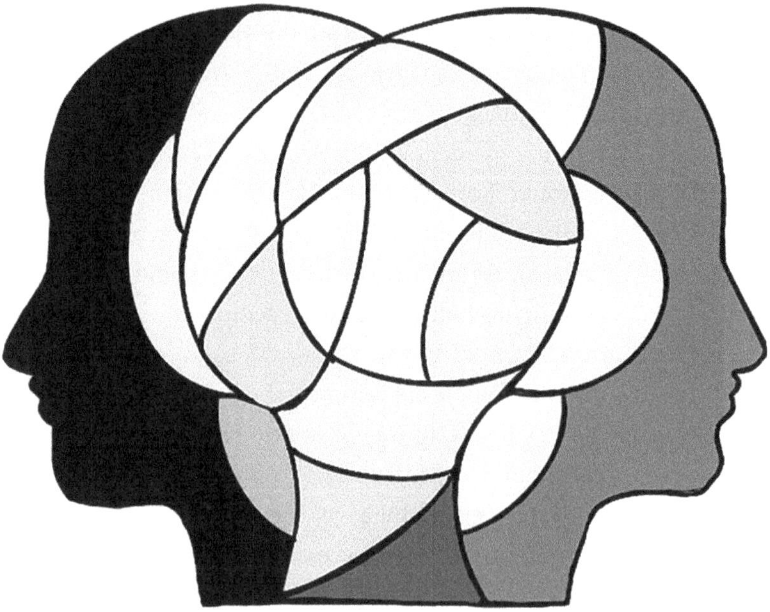

'Social graces' model

Alison Roper-Hall and John B. Burnham, systemic psychotherapists, provide a systemic approach to the way in which we work and think about identity. Systemic psychotherapy is a form of therapy that focuses on relationships and structures rather than focusing on an individual alone, for example families, social networks, organisations within work. Which is where we would usually see problems arise. They developed the 'social graces' model (G, gender and gender identity, geography, generation; R, race, religion; A, age, ability, appearance; C, class, culture, caste; E, education, ethnicity, economics; S, spirituality, sexuality, sexual orientation)[1] to help therapists and people working within the healthcare profession to consider how elements of identity affect themselves and the people who they work with (Burnham 1992, 2012; see also Birdsey and Kustner 2020).

What are the 'social graces'?

Originally, Burnham used 'DISGRRACCE' as an acronym (2012, p.140), to remind him of the main differences to reflect on when working with clients. DISGRRACCE stands for: Disability, I, Sexual, Gender, Race, Religion, Age, Class, Culture and Ethnicity. He used it as a mnemonic to remind him that it would be a 'disgrace' for therapy not to acknowledge our differences. The word 'social', which considers the ways that identities are socially constructed, was added later, to form the 'social graces' model.

The 'social graces' model gives us multiple lenses through which to view identity and to explore where individuals sit within their world. It enables engagement with the ways in which identities are influenced by systemic factors, histories and cultures. This is a strength of the systemic way of thinking.

The 'social graces' acronym is supposed to evolve and expand over time. Reflecting our changing understanding of identity, different 'graces' have been added over time. It is not a fixed list but rather a reflective and flexible tool for therapists or practitioners to use. Used effectively and with awareness of these potential pitfalls, the 'social graces' model offers a reflective and flexible tool for therapists or practitioners to use.

---

1 See, for example, https://norfolklscp.org.uk/media/kfojxutp/5-ggrraaacceeesss.pdf

An easy-to-remember acronym like the 'social graces' model can sometimes be criticised for oversimplifying complex ideas. It risks being used as a 'tick-box' tool, where a therapist or practitioner simply checks off each aspect of identity rather than reflecting deeply on what these aspects mean for the person. The acronym may also unintentionally imply that each 'grace' is separate or independent. In reality, the framework is intended to offer a holistic view of identity. None of the graces stand alone; they are interconnected and together shape the experience of a whole human being.

THE 'SOCIAL GRACES'

Spend 2 minutes looking at the 'social graces' acronym. Now set a timer for 2 minutes, and without looking at the acronym, list as many of the graces as you can remember on a piece of paper. Then, looking at the list you created, answer the following questions:

- How many did you remember?
- Which did you write first?
- Which came towards the end of your list?
- Which did not make your list at all?

This activity can provide valuable insights into the aspects of identity that spark more interest for you. You may, for example, bypass 'geography' as this is not a significant factor in your life, but it may be important for your clients. If you are unaware of this, you may risk overlooking a core part of your client's identity. Alternatively, you may place importance on a particular 'social grace' because of your personal interest or because this feels comfortable for you without full consideration of your client's perspective and experiences (Birdsey and Kustner 2020). Acknowledging this is important and can be discussed in supervision with colleagues who can support you.

We have created a timer that you could use to write in your client's different graces. Invite your client to complete this either independently within the session or with you. You can also try it yourself independently, within clinical supervision or with a mentor.

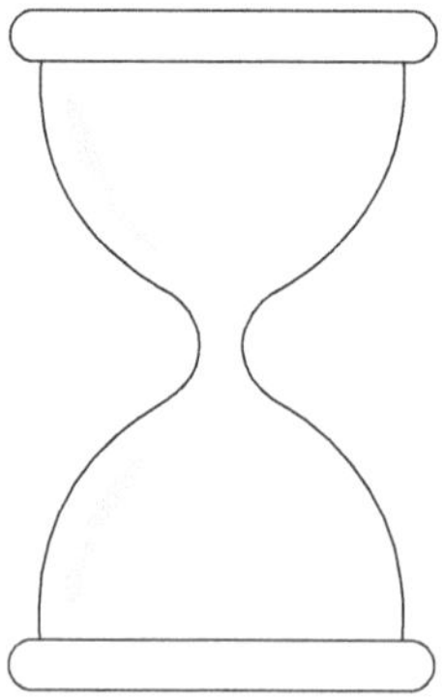

Visible, invisible, voiced and unvoiced 'social graces'

'Social graces' can be visible or invisible, voiced or unvoiced.[2] We may react differently to them because of these factors. Interactions between these can also add further complexity. We can easily make assumptions about a person's identity based on what is unseen (invisible) to us and unvoiced. For example, we may assume a person's gender if they present

2 Burnham (2012) acknowledges that the phrasing of these terms can be problematic as the language of 'seen and unseen, voiced and unvoiced' can be perceived as ableist because people may have disabilities including limited sight, impaired hearing or difficulty speaking.

visually as 'typically' female or male. If their gender identity remains unvoiced, our assumptions will continue. We may make assumptions about a person's religion if they wear a headscarf or about a person's dedication to their religion if they have a visible physical signifier in comparison to someone with religious beliefs whose faith is invisible to us.

We need to tread carefully in relation to what we perceive as 'seen'.

We cannot see a person's class status, but verbal or visual signifiers may present clues. For example, if a person speaks with received pronunciation (RP), you might assume that they are from the middle or upper classes. Some 'social graces', such as race, can be more visible. However, as we know, this is not always clear or simple. Similarly, age can be 'seen', but while we may be able to accurately guess one person's age, we can be wrong in our estimate of another person's age who appears younger or older than they actually are.

In the context of 'unseen social graces', certain disabilities are unseen (often known as 'invisible disabilities'). This may cause distress to the people who experience them because of a lack of understanding that they are disabled and so their needs are not met.

'Social graces' as seen and unseen and voiced and unvoiced are fluid. Their status may change depending on who a person is with and the setting or environment. If a person is comfortable and safe, they may voice their sexuality. They may not share this information if they feel it is not safe or relevant to do so.

Respect clients' agency in choosing whether or not to openly discuss their social graces. Burnham (2012) speaks to the need to practise reflexivity and not to presume the desire of clients to transition from invisible and unvoiced to visible and voiced 'social graces'; he explains that this is not always helpful and can be un-therapeutic.

> **Sarona, a 25-year-old**, was referred to a psychological therapist working in an NHS setting. Sarona was referred for support with anxiety and symptoms of depression. During the initial assessment, the therapist considered culture from the 'social graces' model and how background might inform the client's presentation and experience of distress. NHS clinical guidelines emphasise the importance of

culturally informed care, yet no information about the client's ethnicity or heritage was recorded in the referral or disclosed during intake.

Challenge

The therapist was aware that understanding a client's cultural context can enhance therapeutic engagement and outcomes, particularly in a diverse and multicultural population. However, the client appeared reserved during early sessions and had not volunteered any information about their background. The therapist was concerned that asking directly might feel intrusive or pressured, particularly so early in the therapeutic relationship.

Clinical challenges

While the therapist wanted to practise in a culturally sensitive and informed way, aligning with NHS values of equality, diversity and inclusion, they also recognised that prematurely encouraging disclosure could leave the client feeling exposed or unsafe. This posed a challenge when exploring issues related to identity, belonging and worldview, which may be influenced by cultural heritage.

Outcome

The therapist prioritised building trust and psychological safety over the first few sessions, using open, non-directive language, and validating the client's lived experience without assuming cultural meaning. By not forcing disclosure, the therapist supported the client's autonomy and self-agency. As trust developed, the therapist began to ask more questions, showing further curiosity around the client's cultural background. This led the client to share elements of their cultural background in their own time. This allowed for the client and therapist to reach a more holistic understanding of their challenges and tailoring the intervention and following the client's needs and agency of her sessions.

Reflection

This shows the importance of trauma-informed practice and culturally responsive care within NHS services. It shows that therapists can

> support clients to explore identity and culture as well as upholding NHS values while maintaining choice, respect and autonomy for the client. Cultural awareness is not dependent on immediate disclosure, but when therapists or practitioners create a safe therapeutic space such conversations can naturally emerge.

Bringing the 'social graces' model into therapy

The 'social graces' model allows us to think deeply about someone's background and identity. If it is used as a loose framework, it can give us access to a great deal of information that we may have never considered before because of our own unconscious bias or assumptions. When applying it in a therapeutic context, we have found that the following question, suggested by Burnham (2012), is a useful way to bring the invisible and unvoiced into the room:

> Are there any things that are not immediately obvious about you that you think it is important for me to know?

This question is non-threatening. It gives your client power and choice, and invites them to take the lead with exploring their own identity, sharing what they believe is important for us as therapists or practitioners to know.

Trauma-informed practice

A trauma-informed lens gives therapists and practitioners a more holistic view of their clients' lives. It enables us to understand how trauma can negatively impact someone's life, development, relationships and environment: 'Trauma-informed care is a whole-system approach that recognises, understands and responds to both the prevalence and impact of trauma... in a way that seeks to cause no further harm' (NHS England 2025).

What is trauma?

There are many definitions of trauma. In this book we use the organisation Mind's definition: 'Trauma is when a person experiences a distressing event that they find difficult to cope with.'[3] Trauma can express itself in many ways, including in physical symptoms within our body, such as headaches and tiredness. There can also be internal psychological symptoms, such as anxiety and dissociation.

There are people who are more likely to experience trauma. These include people of colour, the LBGTQIA+ community, those experiencing poverty, those who have been in prison and those who have served in the army.[4] If you are from these marginalised groups it may be difficult to access resources.

Intergenerational and multigenerational trauma

Intergenerational and multigenerational trauma are other types of trauma. In these cases, emotional and psychological harm is passed down from one generation to the next. In the book *Decolonizing Trauma Work*, Renee Linklater states that 'inter/multigenerational trauma is passed on through parental/institutional parenting as well as through bloodlines' (2014, p.35).

Intergenerational and multigenerational trauma is particularly important when working with Indigenous peoples, but is not limited to these communities.

While 'inherited memories' may not be a term all practitioners accept due to a gap in research, the idea that trauma is transmitted across generations is mainly accepted by the scientific community (Cacace and Summers 2024). Epigenetics studies, for example, have identified trauma-linked changes in gene expression in the children and grandchildren of survivors. In her book *The Epigenetics Revolution* (2011), covering the Dutch famine of 1944–45, Nessa Carey explains that prenatal exposure to famine led to altered DNA methylation in children born during the time. It was also shown that the epigenetic changes continued decades later and went on to affect the grandchildren's metabolic health.

---

3 www.mind.org.uk/information-support/types-of-mental-health-problems/trauma/about-trauma

4 www.mind.org.uk/information-support/types-of-mental-health-problems/trauma/about-trauma

Intergenerational trauma

Intergenerational trauma refers to trauma which has been passed down directly from one generation to the other. For example, a parent or caregiver who has lived through a war will have suffered emotional distress and trauma, and this can affect the way in which they may navigate the world and parenting. This can include a parent becoming overprotective with their children, viewing the world as a dangerous place, and therefore passing down their anxieties to their children.

> **AMAL, A 39-YEAR-OLD WOMAN**, originally fled Syria during the civil war. She had witnessed multiple deaths of family members and survived many bombings. Amal spent two years in a refugee camp away from family and friends before migrating to Germany. Amal currently lives in Germany with her husband and her son Tariq, who is five years old.
>
> ### *Psychological impact on Amal*
>
> After resettling in Germany Amal was diagnosed with PTSD (post-traumatic stress disorder) and GAD (generalised anxiety disorder). Amal suffers from nightmares and flashbacks. Due to her prolonged exposure to violence during the war, she has an extreme fear of new places and social settings, as well as loud noises. This is manifested in the following parental behaviours:
>
> - *Overprotectiveness:* Amal never allows her child to visit his friends' houses. He is never allowed to go on school trips. Amal fears that he will be abducted or hurt. Amal only feels comfortable when her child is with her. She struggles not being in close proximity to him.
>
> - *Oversharing:* Amal often shares distressing details of world events and her experiences of the war with Tariq. She often tells her son about how dangerous the world is, leading to Tariq developing an anxious view of the world.

Impact on Tariq

- *Social withdrawal and anxiety:* Tariq often shows signs of separation anxiety, especially when his mother is not within view. Tariq struggles at school, particularly with forming friendships. He exhibits nervous behaviours, such as playing with his hair and nail biting.

- *Lack of autonomy:* Tariq struggles when needing to make decisions. He often gets overwhelmed and finds decision-making difficult. He also struggles with being alone and often needs a teacher with him when starting tasks.

- *Anxieties and fears:* Tariq has internalised his mother's fears and views the world as a dangerous place. Like his mother, he is also afraid of loud noises. Although Tariq does not have first-hand experience of war, he demonstrates comparable behaviours to children who have lived through war.

This shows the impact of intergenerational trauma: even though Tariq did not witness the war directly, he is still impacted by the emotionally intense and anxious environment that he is growing up and lives in.

Multigenerational trauma

Multigenerational or transgenerational trauma is trauma that has been transmitted through several generations. Multigenerational trauma can be spread not just from a parent but via an entire lineage of people. This unresolved trauma, passed from one generation to the next, can continue cycles of systemic oppression and difficulties. For example, colonisation, which leads to the forced displacement of Indigenous peoples and their communities, impacts multiple generations. The cumulative effects of colonisation build over time, and its effects on many aspects of life, including identity, continue across generations. It directly contributes to mental health difficulties and reinforces systemic oppressions, such as socioeconomic hardships.

Stefan is a 42-year-old man who was born and raised in an isolated Roma settlement. His family has been living in these settlements for generations, facing intense discrimination and poverty. Stefan's father and grandfather often share their memories of being chased out of neighbourhoods and towns by people, including the police. This has created a sense of fear and instability within the family. Stefan has two children, and is anxious and concerned about their future. He often worries about discrimination and segregation within the school environment.

Stefan works in informal labour jobs. He struggles to provide for his family and relies on government support. However, this support is never enough, and Stefan cannot break the financial insecurity cycle. He has noticed that his children show signs of anxiety. They have mentioned that they feel different to and isolated from the non-Roma students at school.

Stefan's mental health struggles

- Stefan struggles with anxiety and low moods. He has felt this way ever since he was a young boy. Stefan has never been able to break the social-economic trap created through historical and systemic discrimination.
- Stefan often has sleepless nights and nightmares.

Stefan's children's mental health struggles

- Symptoms of anxiety and stress.
- A sense of isolation and exclusion.

This shows how transgenerational trauma is passed on. The Roma community has experienced centuries of ongoing discrimination, displacement, systemic oppression, enslavement and persecution. This has contributed to a legacy of transgenerational trauma that has affected people's mental health and created socioeconomic marginalisation, cultural loss and identity struggles.

Adverse childhood experiences

Adverse childhood experiences, a term referring to stressful and potential traumatic events in early life, are often known by the acronym ACEs. The World Health Organization (WHO) lists the following as ACEs: as 'multiple types of abuse; neglect; violence between parents or caregivers; other kinds of serious household dysfunction such as alcohol and substance abuse; and peer, community and collective violence' (2018).

ACEs affect a child's physical and emotional health as well as their development. An awareness of their impact can enable greater understanding of someone's experience of trauma. While an awareness of ACEs can support creative work on identity, we must avoid 're-traumatisation' – when a person experiences their trauma again, reliving emotions or physical feelings that were experienced at the time of the traumatic experience. Any therapist or practitioner discussing traumatic experiences with clients must be aware of how to sensitively hold the emotions and feelings that may arise (see, for example, NHS England 2025).

When using the activities in this book, it is essential to take a reflective, trauma-informed approach to limit the potential risk of re-traumatisation and harm.

What is trauma-informed practice?

Trauma-informed practices have developed from several different fields including social care, health organisations and psychological therapies. There are six key principles of trauma-informed practice (Office for Health Improvements & Disparities 2022):

- *Safety:* Safety within the organisation in which you work is also key. You do not sit in isolation; you represent who and where you work.

- *Choice:* The choice for the client to say they are not ready to explore this part of themselves in your working relationship is especially important in avoiding re-traumatisation.

- *Trustworthiness:* Trustworthiness within the organisation relates to the practitioner working with the client being clear on what they are doing and why, and saying what they will do in order to create trust between the client and organisation.

- *Collaboration:* Perhaps you are asking your client to consider parts of themselves they are not yet ready to disclose. It's important to make this process collaborative by asking them what they need, considering the organisation and your ability to meet those needs, working alongside, and not *doing to.*

- *Empowerment:* The client needs to feel empowered to have a choice around whether they would like to partake in these activities and to make their own decisions. Empowerment refers to supporting your client to make decisions about their care by actively listening and validating their feelings.

- *Cultural consideration:* We must practise cultural consideration by being aware of stereotyping, biases and making assumptions towards our clients when thinking about identity. Part of being human is to stereotype others as a way of predicting behaviour and keeping ourselves safe. However, this is unhelpful behaviour when working with a client's identity, and something we need to develop an awareness of as therapists and practitioners. We are naturally biased towards people who look like ourselves and those who are from similar areas or backgrounds, so it is vital to create an awareness around this in order to avoid entrenching bias and its effects.

Some questions for discussing trauma and identity in a therapeutic context

Recognising that trauma is rooted in multiple intersecting elements of a person's identity allows for a more nuanced approach to therapy. The following questions can help guide the therapist or practitioner through a compassionate approach:

- Can you identify a time when you felt misunderstood or unseen because of an aspect of your identity?
- Have certain experiences shaped the way you feel in different spaces?
- In what spaces do you feel safe or unsafe?
- What does safety mean to you? What does it look like?
- Are there parts of your identity or culture that have changed or evolved over time?

If you would rather not go into this right now, we can pause and come back to this later. It's okay if the questions feel complex – identity is layered and dynamic. Take as much time as you need.

These questions aim to help you understand your client better, by recognising that systems of oppression, lived experiences and intersectionality impact how we navigate the world. They are here to guide and not pressurise the client to recount trauma or disclose anything they are not ready to.

Bringing a trauma-informed lens into therapy

We encourage therapists and practitioners to engage with these activities using trauma-informed principles. This will look different depending on your practice and setting, but fundamentally it requires providing safety, choice, trust, collaboration, empowerment and cultural consideration. A way of effectively applying this approach when using an activity may be to ask yourself whether you and your client have built a safe relationship. Consider the following:

- Has your client already communicated that they feel safe within the therapeutic relationship?
- What would make your client feel safe when exploring challenging parts of their identity?
- What does safety mean to your client, and how would they know that they feel safe?

You need to be explicit in your aims and rationale when introducing an activity, and communicate this in a way that feels collaborative and safe to your client. Ask yourself:

- Is your client able to say 'no' to you?
- Does your client have other ways of saying 'no' if they don't feel able to verbalise this?
- Are you giving your client time to think about the activity before introducing it?

If your answers to these questions are 'no', then you are in danger of potentially re-traumatising your client. Your client needs to feel empowered to choose whether or not they would like to partake in the activities. The choice for them to say they are not ready to explore this part of themselves in your working relationship is very important in keeping them feeling empowered and maintaining a sense of agency within the therapeutic intervention. It's important to work collaboratively, to ask your client what they need, to consider the organisational context, and to assess your ability to meet those needs. By actively listening to your client and validating their feelings, they will feel supported to make decisions about their care. This will create a sense of empowerment rather than re-traumatisation.

Reflective and responsive practice

The activities in this book engage with the complex and sensitive subject of intersectional identity. It is therefore important to monitor clients' responses to activities and to attune to their needs, as you would in your usual therapeutic session. Your client may experience a fear response or dissociative state, which you must respond and adapt to throughout an activity, bringing it to an end if appropriate. People may respond to an activity in unpredictable or surprising ways, with an inability to consciously locate where this comes from. They may not carry these feelings within their conscious brain; it may be a trauma response, particularly in response to discrimination based on intersecting aspects of identity. Your client may have experienced some form of trauma which may, in turn, present during the therapeutic interaction. When working with trauma, it is important to be aware of the fight, flight, fear or fawn trauma responses.

What to look out for in fight, flight, fear or fawn trauma responses

- A fight response may look like: frustration, anger, defensiveness or control.
- A flight response may look like: anxiety or an avoidance of answering questions.
- A fear response may look like: dissociation, numbness or an inability to speak.
- A fawn response may look like: people-pleasing or co-dependency.

These responses are normal reactions to overwhelming experiences such as childhood trauma or ongoing trauma. They are ultimately there to protect our clients from harm. If you notice any of these responses in the session you must pause, react and support your client safely. A trauma-informed therapist will help the client recognise and name their survival responses, offering them some psychoeducation on the way our nervous systems try to protect us with these bodily responses.

Resmaa Menakem (2021) writes about the 'soul nerve' as the nerve that feels and receives the trauma response but that is also responsible for calming the body afterwards. The soul nerve is also known as the polyvagal nervous system; this feels your emotions and is connected to every part of the body except the thinking brain. It can be key in calming your body down after experiencing heightened emotions. Identity work and trauma-informed practice aim to strengthen the soul nerve, bringing the client to a place of safety, and supporting their emotional and physical experiences.

CHAPTER 2

Identity and Culture

What do we mean by identity and culture? In this chapter, we investigate the meanings of identity and culture and the different facets of culture and identity work. We explore how we can bring identity and culture into therapeutic work to develop inclusive anti-discriminatory and anti-oppressive practice, and we attempt to decolonise therapeutic interventions.

What is identity and culture?

The word 'identity' comes from the Latin *identitas*, meaning 'sameness'. Identity refers to the characteristics and traits of a person or group of people, including personal attributes such as gender, sexuality, age and ethnicity. We have decided to define 'culture' as set beliefs, societies, rituals and linguistics that are learned and transmitted across generations. Erik Erikson, a German-American psychoanalyst and psychologist, was one of the first people to integrate the term 'identity' into therapy, and one of the only psychoanalysts and psychologists who considered sociological systems when thinking about clients or patients. The term 'identity', along with Erikson's theories on identity, was first introduced in his book *Childhood and Society* (1950/1995).

Erikson's theory of identity

Erikson explores the myriad ways in which we each come to construct a sense of self, drawing on how we are socialised during our formative years, and how environments can contour behavioural patterns, subsequently informing the ways identities are sustained through a set of specific cultural frameworks. Erikson calls this 'ego identity': built on a conscious sense of self through social interaction. He posited that a robust sense of self is constructed between modes of social interaction and our emotional self. Within this process, he observed the significant function of 'locales', defined as the different contexts, settings and environments in which someone's psychological experiences and behaviours are shaped. As locales shift, so does the interpersonal. Locales include not just physical spaces but also cultural, social and emotional environments.

Two types of locales shape a person's psychological experiences:

- *Physical locales* are tangible environments, such as where a person lives, spends most of their time or works. They affect a person's psychological development and mental health, depending on factors such as safety and access to resources. For example, a child living in a conflict zone will not have the same advantages (such as a safe physical living environment) as, say, a child living in London.

- *Social locales* are the social environments, such as friends, family, teachers and colleagues, with whom a person interacts. The quality of our social locales has a significant effect on our psychological experience and development. Nurturing, caring and understanding friends, family, teachers and colleagues can enhance feelings of belonging.

Transformations to a person's psychological experience can be made by adjusting the catalogue of personhood, such as social roles, cultural expectations and/or relational identities, which forthcoming generations come to inherit. We can adjust these catalogues within society by redefining a person's psychological experience and broadening our understanding of what it means to be human. We have already seen this take place within feminist movements and the LGBTQIA+ communities, and within social, cultural and political spaces that challenge the status quo. We have seen how this has profoundly shifted the way we see sexuality and gender within the UK, for example expanding the 'catalogue' for future generations by validating non-heteronormative identities and the fluidity of gender roles.

Erikson's theory outlines eight stages of psychosocial development, from infancy to older adulthood. The theory postulates that our basic needs from infancy to older adulthood need to be met. If our emotional needs are satisfied by our social environment, this helps to feed our sense of autonomy. Imagine a child at the school-age stage of Erikson's theory, the time when a child is building their self-competence. They are beginning to socialise and trying out activities such as art, music and sport. What happens if that child is told they cannot participate or should not be interested in certain subjects?

Consider a child with a physical disability who wants to participate in school sports but is told they cannot due to their disability. Instead of being offered an alternative activity that meets their needs and builds their confidence, they are excluded entirely. This exclusion may create a belief that they are incapable of participating in sports, eventually generalising this perception to other areas of life. Without opportunities for encouragement or involvement, the child might internalise a sense of inadequacy. Over time, this belief can solidify, causing the child to feel inferior and doubt their abilities.

If a child's interests are not facilitated and they are unable to participate and be curious around their surroundings and environments, this could lead to difficulties in forming a cohesive identity. When needs are met and encouraged at each stage, according to Erikson, a person can build a strong sense of self. A person with a strong sense of self can endure change and challenges because of this. Therefore, building a child's resilience, confidence and interests, and bringing more of their identity and culture into relationships, is important for the development of a strong sense of self.

The relationship between identity and culture is a dynamic one, constantly in flux and changing. Identity and culture are constantly interacting together and overlapping with one another. So how can we facilitate the development of a strong sense of self when our needs have not been met? Typically, our sense of self is affected when we are met with challenges between cultural normative systems, their expectations and our personal identity.

Tajfel's social identity theory

Henri Tajfel, who played a significant role in the development of social psychology in Europe, researched intergroup behaviour and its influence on identity. Tajfel's first-hand experiences of discrimination and prejudice during the Second World War helped to shape his interests around identity and discrimination. He was a prisoner of war and wrestled with hiding his own Jewish identity and telling his capturers the truth that he was Jewish while knowing that this could threaten his life. He did eventually choose to disclose his Jewish identity to his capturers, risking death. Tajfel's struggles were rooted in discrimination, oppression and social categorisation. His life experiences, particularly his survival from the Holocaust and the death of his family, deeply influenced his subsequent research.

Tajfel proposed that 'identity' is developed by the acceptance and membership of certain groups. As humans, we do not do well with uncertainty. One way in which we can deal with uncertainties, such as cultural uncertainty, is by grouping.

Tajfel *et al.* (1971) conducted an experiment where people were grouped at random. Grouping was not built on any conflict, and nor was there any importance placed on the group members' personalities and shared experiences, meaning there was no shared group identity. The purpose was to see if grouping people at random was enough to form a shared group identity. Would the group show a preference towards the members of the group they were randomly selected to be in? As Tajfel predicted, the experiment showed that the group members favoured their assigned group, showing in-group favouritism and out-group discrimination. This shows us the power of labelling and grouping. Grouping people and labelling can influence our decision-making, dominance, privileges and oppressions. Grouping people provides a sense of order.

If the groups we are part of are under attack, we begin to feel a direct attack ourselves.

A group's identity significantly shapes and influences human behaviour. It provides a sense of belonging and understanding through shared life experiences with fellow members, especially when we have chosen what group to be part of.

When individuals are placed into an 'outsider group' without choosing to be part of it, both the individual and the group as a whole are impacted. Yet, this shared exclusion can also strengthen the bond within the outsider group. The group can form a sense of solidarity as they find common ground in their shared experiences.

Bringing culture into therapy

To bring culture and identity into therapeutic work, we must first acknowledge that our identity and culture do not start or begin with *therapist* and *client*. Both therapist and client carry their own long-standing history as well as historical legacies, such as colonialism and slavery, where power has played a role in historical events.

Therapists and clients do not only meet each other in the room, but they also bring with them the history of their ancestors and their traumas. Therefore, when bringing culture into therapy, therapists and clients are asked to think about their own positions with power within their own narratives. Both therapist and client constantly bounce back and forth, from being the *most powerful* and the *most powerless* person. Inviting clients to offer us insights into their cultural knowledge through collaboration will help to decolonise therapy, move away from Eurocentric theories and build new ways of working.

To engage with culture in therapy, the therapist should look at a client's individual context: for example, where a client fits into social, political and structural systems. The therapist should pay attention to a client's history, colonial or post-colonial history, race, ethnicity, religion and/or other intersections that define culture and how it plays into the client's systems. To take a holistic approach to culture, therapists need to consider their positions and those of their clients within systems, whether economical, familial or historical. Viewing systems through the lens of culture can encourage conversations within the therapeutic relationship. Reflecting on clients and therapists' individual experiences of systems can offer an insight into shared experiences and create space for exploring different experiences. Providing culturally appropriate care to clients may help increase a better response to therapy for Indigenous or minoritised communities, for example.

Culture follows patterns, customs and rituals according to which a person experiences the world they are part of. Keeping culture at the forefront of a client's therapeutic journey promotes authenticity. Therapists incorporating culture into therapy should engage with and be mindful of the following:

- *Cultural humility:* This involves recognising and acknowledging our own cultural biases. The therapist or practitioner should approach the therapeutic relationship as a collaborative partnership in which both parties actively contribute. This requires the therapist to identify their own limitations within the therapeutic process, which is an essential process for effective practice. By recognising these limitations, therapists can ensure they provide the best possible support to their clients. At times, it may be appropriate to refer a client to a more suitable therapeutic intervention or to another professional who can offer more specialist care. This approach not only enhances the quality of care but also reduces the risk of harm to the client. For example, a client may experience setbacks in their therapeutic journey if the therapist fails to understand the client's unique experiences due to limitations in their own practice. As therapists, it is our responsibility to recognise our boundaries and operate within our scope of competence.

- *Scope of competence:* This is where our expertise lies. Adhering to this scope helps maintain the integrity of our profession. It is also important to inform clients about our specific areas of knowledge and the limits of our practice. By committing to ongoing professional development and actively addressing our limitations, we can expand our knowledge and continue to provide high-quality care.

- *Cultural sensitivity:* This is awareness of a client's culture and approaching this sensitively and respectfully, while simultaneously adhering to ethical guidelines and professional standards. We can incorporate cultural sensitivity within a therapeutic intervention with a client by asking them open-ended questions – for example, 'Do you believe that your religion plays a role in the way you view your mental health and wellbeing?'

- *Cultural relativism:* This is the idea that cultures and people should be understood within their own cultural context. People should not be evaluated. There is no universal standard that would allow us to measure a person or their culture. Instead, cultures and people should be understood within their own culture or cultural context rather than evaluated based on a model of culture and a single objective standard which does not exist. For example, there is no value in evaluating Middle Eastern culture using the standards of British culture. Embracing other cultural values can lead to a discipline which opposes discrimination and is committed to the pursuit of social justice and authenticity within our work with our clients.

- *Generalisations:* These happen all the time and can occur within our intimate relationships or with strangers, clients and other professionals we communicate with. For example, a therapist may respond to a client who has suffered a bereavement by saying 'I'm sorry for your loss'. This generalisation assumes that the client is feeling sadness with respect to the bereavement. Although this assumption may be true, death is actually celebrated in some cultures and heritages. Alternatively, for some bereaved people their relationship with the deceased was complex or compromised and, for them, sadness is not the emotion they may want to be exploring in therapy.

Recognising cultural difference in therapy

The field of therapy is often seen as a profession that is culturally sensitive, meaning that it strives to understand people and their cultural differences, where therapists navigate difference with awareness, understanding and respect. As therapists and practitioners, therefore, we must attempt to become comfortable with cultural difference and the challenges we face within the difference. A common mistake is to think cultural sensitivity means not asking about a client's cultural differences. This can hinder therapeutic work because avoiding discussion on cultural identity can lead to misunderstandings and unspoken issues not being explored. In this chapter, we have provided an example of cultural difference viewed through the lens of race. However, cultural difference is by no means limited to racial difference; identity and culture work is complex and multifaceted.

Cultural similarities and differences in beliefs, power dynamics and communication, for example, can affect the way in which a therapist meaningfully connects to a client, and vice versa. In the case of cultural similarities, if a client from India has an Indian clinician they may have an understanding of Indian culture that a clinician from another country may not have. This may enable a sense of shared cultural understanding.

However, therapeutic relationships are complex and this doesn't mean that it is better to see a therapist with a similar cultural background. While it is important for therapists to bring difference and similarities into the therapeutic space, an overemphasis on difference can create distance between the therapist and client. This distance can cause the client to feel 'othered'. This is why approaching difference with curiosity, observation, openness and balance is pivotal. As therapists and mental health practitioners our differences may also interfere with therapeutic goals. Therapeutic goals should always include an in-depth analysis of a client's history and current situation as well as goals that have been co-produced with the client.

The same can be said about an overemphasis on similarities within a therapeutic relationship. Kristina is a British Cypriot, working-class, female art psychotherapist. However, this does not mean that her life experiences would be the same as another Cypriot woman living in the UK, or that she is an expert on the Cypriot identity. As we are aware, identity and culture are more nuanced than that. We may share similarities with other people, depending on our race, religion or sexuality, but human beings are never the same. Therefore, overemphasising similarities can lead to a therapist or practitioner overlooking other aspects of a client's experience, causing the client to feel invisible and dismissed.

Unconscious bias

In the context of similarities and differences, it is important to acknowledge unconscious bias. This term refers to the automatic response and attitude a person has towards another person based on characteristics such as race, heritage, age, gender and sexual orientation. These biases can operate outside of our conscious awareness, but they affect and influence our choices and decisions. They can begin from an early age and be passed to us via familial beliefs, friendships, interests, our environment, and through the media.

There can be an assumption that we have limited control of our unconscious biases, but this is not the case. We can learn new ways to identify and even deal with our unconscious biases and prejudices before they can cause harm.

At times, our unconscious biases can influence our automatic reactions. We may be in a state of fear without time to process or reason. The amygdala, which is located within the temporal lobes of the brain, is responsible for the way in which we respond to threat. Usually, it involves the connection between emotion and memory. Therefore, if we are reacting to another person as a threat or with fear, this usually means that our amygdala is activated. If something or someone feels unknown or unfamiliar, then this can simultaneously ignite our prejudices, formed by stereotypes, and affect the way in which we interact and respond to them.

Pragya Agarwal, in her book *Sway: Unravelling Unconscious Bias* (2021), explains that we often form stereotypes based on social categorisation. These stereotypes often occur 'spontaneously', and as Tajfel expressed, we then assign people into groups because of them. We are more likely to interact with people who form part of our own membership groups and respond to others with a stereotypical judgement. Agarwal further explores that this is particularly obvious within male and female gender bias.

It feels very natural to be drawn to people who look like us, sound like us or share similar interests to us. This can provide an exchange of positive experiences, especially when similarities can offer a sense of belonging. If we are forming relationships around similarities, this can create deep connections, although for the person who does not match our similarities, we can expect them to have a negative experience with unconscious bias. Unconscious bias impacts the therapeutic relationship as it can subtly influence a therapist or practitioner's therapeutic intervention. For example, a therapist or practitioner may downplay a client's experience if it does not align with their own worldview.

How may unconscious bias show up in the therapy room?

- Misdiagnosing or overdiagnosing clients from marginalised groups: If a therapist is unfamiliar with how certain cultures may exhibit distress, this can cause misdiagnosis or overdiagnosis.

- Assumptions: A therapist or practitioner may assume a client from a certain racial group or heritage has specific values or struggles, and this is the same for everyone in this group.

Race as a cultural difference

Creating a dialogue with our clients around race as a cultural difference can offer a dynamic experience by influencing both therapist and client to learn about the other's lived experience. This exchange can foster growth, understanding and change, with new beginnings being formed while navigating cultural difference. In relation to the dialogue around race, it is important that we understand that race should be used as a context marker rather than a visual characteristic. Race as a cultural difference does not have a fixed position and varies with each individual, depending on their encounters (Campbell 2012, p.42).

The works of poet and educator Claudia Rankine have remodelled the way in which we, the authors, think and talk about race. In Rankine's book *Just Us* (2020), she explores her subjective experiences with race and the dynamics of racial interactions. Rankine simultaneously explores the discomfort and ease within her own relationships around sameness and difference. As a Black woman married to a white man, and who also has a good friend who is white, for Rankine, it seemed impossible to stay focused on sameness within relationships. She says: '...it is in fact my friend's ability to grasp and hold our differences that creates both our facility with each other and our antagonisms. But why, even for a second, translate ease with each other into a state of sameness?' (2020, p.189).

Rankine communicates to us that difference can stir up hostility between people. This hostility or tension should not be avoided. Therapists and practitioners can find this challenging when working with a client therapeutically, particularly when practising cultural sensitivity. In fact, we should become conscious of our differences so that we do not become passive with our clients. Passivity within the therapeutic relationship can cause distance, causing the therapist and client's identity to disappear. Instead, what may be beneficial is to open conversation around difference by using reflection as a means for understanding.

Amina, a Black woman in her early 30s, has started seeing a white female therapist in her 40s. Amina started therapy to explore workplace stress, anxiety and her sense of not being 'seen' in predominately white spaces.

The early sessions

Amina often hesitates before sharing with her therapist her frustrations with her colleagues. She avoids naming these feelings and experiences as being racially charged. Amina's therapist provides a safe space for Amina to explore her feelings; she always responds with empathy and has suggested coping tools to help with her frustrations with her co-workers' actions (which she is unaware Amina feels are racially charged). Amina shows up regularly, but does not seem to be fully engaged within her sessions, and sometimes seems distant.

Supervision

The therapist takes the issue of Amina's lack of engagement to supervision. Her supervisor asks her to practise reflexivity and consider her own whiteness, what this may represent in terms of positions of power and privilege, and how this might be influencing the therapeutic relationship. The therapist explores her own avoidance of asking Amina questions around race and identity, and how this avoidance is having an impact on Amina's progress in therapy by not interrogating the cause of her work-related distress.

Turning point session

In a later session, the therapist gently encourages and introduces reflection within the sessions. She names that sometimes cultural differences can feel difficult to talk about within therapy, especially differences around race, when the therapist and client come from different backgrounds. The therapist reinstates that these sessions need to feel safe for Amina to bring her whole self, including differences, into the sessions. Amina feels seen and validated by this, and expresses that she has found it difficult to bring these experiences into therapy without feeling that she needs to overexplain her experiences. This session is a turning point for Amina, as she begins to explore her internalised experiences with the therapist now that the therapist has made room for difference to be explored.

If our differences are left unspoken, we risk losing understanding of the dynamics of the therapeutic relationship. Keeping cultural sensitivity in mind, we can move into a space of reflection with the client. Reflection can enable connection with the other. As stated by Peter Rober: 'Besides cultural difference, there is also a shared humanity that can arise out of the particular moment...' (Rober 2012: foreword).

Bringing an awareness of race as a cultural difference into therapy

The following approaches and qualities can help to facilitate a trusting therapeutic relationship. They can also encourage dialogue around race and difference within therapy, and enable therapists to challenge the status quo:

- *Creating a safe space:* Facilitating a warm, empathetic space that acknowledges and validates a client's lived experience.

- *Listening:* Mutual listening, not listening to respond but listening to understand a client's position in the world. Taking turns to communicate is an important way to understand what race and cultural difference means to different people.

- *Maintaining curiosity:* The therapist must maintain curiosity throughout their work with their clients. This supports the development of a true, authentic connection with a client, and can also bring dual understanding for both the client and therapist. It shows that life is multidimensional and complex, and that someone's experience with culture is not linear. A person does not fall into one category of culture but many.

- *Ensuring solidarity:* Empathy is important for the therapeutic relationship, and so is solidarity. For example, if a therapist describes themselves as anti-racist, then perhaps they should think about how they show this inside and outside the therapeutic room. Even when our clients are not there and do not know about the work we are doing outside of therapy, it is important to help dismantle certain systemic systems, approaches and beliefs. This encourages cultural change within organisations. You can show your solidarity by signing up to courses on culture and identity, further reading and research, and even having uncomfortable conversations to ensure clients' voices are being heard.

- *Creating an intersubjective space:* This is a conscious process between the therapist and client. The process can be both verbal and non-verbal, for example the positioning of one's body within the therapeutic room and the use of body language. Intersubjectivity, for many cultures, does not require verbal communication but is felt within the body, a form of connection and even softening to someone's body. This is facilitated by learning more about the other through joint participation. Intersubjectivity – the shared and mutual understanding that emerges between two or more individuals during an encounter – can be achieved with play, creativity and curiosity during therapeutic interventions.

- *Adapting and being flexible:* The therapist may need to adapt their sessions around conversations of difference, for example needing to bring these conversations back into the space the following week. The idea is that difference should be woven into therapy. By prioritising reflection and processing with a client, there may be a need to suggest that sometimes the therapist and client may need to revisit or take a break from certain discussions, to come back at a later date, together, to develop further dialogue around difference. This should be a joint conversation, and the client should always be involved in the planning and discussions.

Prompts to encourage conversations around difference

- Can you share what difference means to you?
- What is one thing you wish others understood about you and your identity?
- Have you ever felt 'othered' by difference?
- Are there ways you still feel connected to others regardless of difference?
- What strengths have come from difference? Please share any personal experiences, if you feel comfortable.
- What do you need in order to share your experience around difference?
- What does difference look like, smell like and taste like for you?

We chose to focus on race to explore cultural difference within therapy, but difference can show up in the room in many ways. For example, difference can be religion, gender, sexuality, disability, class, fertility, geography and/or English as a second language. Therapists can adapt these explorative dialogue narratives, to encourage conversations for all difference that enters the room. With basic trust and a shared curiosity of the other, we can override some of the mistrust we have built for survival.

Developing reflexivity within therapy

Systemic psychotherapy has played a significant role in placing culture at the forefront of client work. The term 'reflexivity' is increasingly used within the helping professions, referring to the ability to critically examine and reflect on our own beliefs, values, cultural influences and biases, as well as the impact these have on interactions with individuals from different cultural backgrounds than our own. In therapy, reflexivity specifically pertains to the therapist's or practitioner's capacity to reflect on their own thoughts, experiences, biases and emotions when working with clients. This practice is especially crucial when engaging with clients from diverse cultural contexts.

Traditionally, many therapists have adhered to a non-judgemental stance, a concept central to person-centred therapy and humanistic psychology, as developed by Carl Rogers (1961). This approach fosters a safe, trusting therapeutic relationship, creating an environment where clients feel encouraged to embark on a safe therapeutic journey and explore themselves. While human nature can make maintaining a non-judgemental attitude challenging, reflexivity offers therapists the tools to recognise and challenge their own biases, ensuring they remain present and open in their work with clients.

How can reflexivity improve therapeutic relationships?

Here are some examples of obstacles in therapeutic relationships and suggestions of how reflexivity can support work with clients.

The therapist or practitioner's identity

This is often missing in the therapeutic discourse. Both the therapist or practitioner and the client or groups come with their own histories and power positions. Bringing the therapist's or practitioner's identity into the relationship can help everyone involved to understand what is happening in the relational dynamic of therapist or practitioner and client. Traditionally, therapy or therapeutic interventions focus solely on the client's identity. This can make identity and culture work more difficult to explore, as it almost implies the therapist or practitioner does not have an identity. This becomes an issue especially when we are attempting to address power and privileges or differences and similarities within a therapeutic session. Naming differences and similarities comes with acknowledging the therapist's identity from the outset.

How or where do we bring the therapist or practitioner's identity into the therapeutic relationship?

- *In clinical supervision:* By bringing the therapist's or practitioner's identity into clinical supervision, we make room for it and acknowledge the transference and countertransference of the relationship. This process allows for the exploration of identity and any biases, which can be reflected on and addressed within a safe and confidential space.

- *During therapy or therapeutic interventions:* Sharing elements of your identity with your client can normalise their challenges and struggles. Moreover, appropriate self-disclosure can benefit a client by enhancing the client's experience of therapy and creating a stronger, more authentic therapeutic relationship.

Positions of power in therapeutic alliance

Therapists or practitioners must notice their own power positions that they hold within the therapeutic relationship and their positions within social systems. Our clients meet with us during the most vulnerable times of their lives, so it is important to understand power. Acknowledging the power dynamics within the therapeutic relationship may help with rapport between the client and therapist or practitioner. It will also help to build safety and trust within the relationship. Here is a sentence you could use with a client to acknowledge power imbalances (please adjust the language in your own way so it feels authentic for you):

> I am aware that, as your therapist [or insert job title], I hold a position of power in this space, and this can create power imbalances within our relationship. I would like to make sure that during our time together, you feel heard, respected and empowered to share openly with me. If at any point you feel uncomfortable or that the balance isn't right, please let me know.

Blind spots

Psychological blind spots refer to the areas in which a therapist or practitioner lacks awareness or insight of a client's experience. Blind spots occur all the time. As therapists or practitioners and humans, we often miss or are unable to understand aspects of our clients' identities because we are shaped by our own life experiences. One way in which blind spots occur in therapeutic relationships is when we are too fixed on one approach or framework when working with our clients. This rigid way of working does not allow for adaptations to the client's needs.

How do we address blind spots in therapeutic relationships?

- *Feedback:* One way to address blind spots is with feedback from other professionals and the client. Clinical supervision and peer supervision can be positive in addressing the therapeutic relationship and a client's needs. Receiving feedback within these spaces can help with the identification of blind spots and increase awareness. Moreover, encouraging a client to provide the therapist or practitioner with feedback on the intervention and therapeutic process is important to be able to hear the client's experience. It also enables clients to raise any concerns they may have about the therapeutic process. For example, you could ask a client the following questions at the end of one of the activities in Part 2 of the book:
  - Is there anything you feel is missing from these sessions?
  - Is there anything you would like to discuss more about identity and culture within our sessions?
  - How could I adapt our session to meet your needs?
  - How was today's session for you? Is there anything you would like more of or less of?

- *Seeing difference:* If a therapist perceives everybody as sharing a universal culture and has limited awareness of their own cultural experiences, privileges and oppressions, they risk losing the potential for understanding their clients, and instead increase the likelihood of misunderstandings.

By therapists or practitioners using reflexivity in therapy or therapeutic interventions and turning inward, examining themselves, they can gain valuable insights into another person's perspective. Psychotherapy and epistemology intersect in significant ways, particularly in how therapists conceptualise knowledge. For instance, when therapists or practitioners adopt a socially constructed view of knowledge, it can shape the client's narrative. This can even be drawn down to the frameworks a therapist or practitioner is basing their interventions on. Maintaining conscious awareness of this influence is crucial, as it allows therapists or practitioners to navigate its use thoughtfully within the therapeutic encounter.

Reflexivity and epistemological awareness invite therapists to critically examine their own biases and epistemic stance, enabling them to better understand how their views on knowledge, culture and identity might impact the therapeutic relationship. The Western approach to mental health particularly tends to isolate the individual and their lived experience. In this model, academic knowledge and treatments based on academic knowledge take precedence over different approaches from other regions, cultures and traditions.

Capitalism and discrimination within therapy

We believe that it is vital to address capitalism in the context of therapy. Looking at therapy via a capitalist critique enables an understanding of the context in which it operates, especially within the West. By understanding the effects of capitalism and its oppressive structures, this helps us as therapists or practitioners to understand and challenge the individualistic approach that capitalism often promotes within therapy, and therefore our therapeutic interventions.

Sigmund Freud often referred to the 'inner world' of the client as the internal psychological states of a person, such as their unconscious desires and conflicts (1915/1957). He suggests that these unconscious desires and conflicts are what shape us as people and influence our behaviours and actions. Freud believed that by exploring a client's internal world and psyche, a client would reach a better understanding of themselves. Many psychodynamic psychotherapists still place much of their therapeutic interventions and reasonings on Freud and Carl Jung's literature (on Jung, see Stevens 1994). Both Freud and Jung believed that much of our outer expressions were due to our inner desires from the psyche. However, the same importance is not placed on our clients' external environments or to understanding how our clients' actions may be a form of survival to their external environments.

Modern-day society has been shaped by hundreds of years of industrial capitalism. In the 21st century, capitalism is still being critiqued for widening the gap between the rich and poor. In the UK, capitalism is still the governing economic system. The pursuit of profit is embedded within this economic system, leading to burnout and the exploitation of people and natural resources. At the time of writing, we continue to experience rising living costs, including energy bill increases and high mortgage interest rates, all while wages for the average person remain stagnant.

The relationship between therapy and capitalism has been a complicated one, ever since their inception. Within Western culture, there is an underlying assumption that individuals have the freedom to explore their desires and interests in daily life. However, from birth, we live within a system that assigns us birth certificates and passports, and grants us access to educational institutions, future job prospects and the freedom to travel. These systems are intended to provide opportunities for personal and professional growth, including employment and even the hope of securing a home, thereby contributing to individual and regional economic prosperity. However, these systems also fall short. For example, refugees may lack access to official identity documents, making their ability to access basic systems like education and housing challenging. This leaves them more vulnerable and at greater risk of exploitation. Moreover, trans and non-binary people often will face bureaucratic and legal challenges when they're attempting to update their gender. The importance of exploring these systems and identity simultaneously acknowledges that there is no such thing as just the individual. Exploring capitalism in therapy is important because it shapes nearly every aspect of our lives. Due to this, capitalism also affects our mental health, our relationships and our accessibility to care.

Capitalism's influence on identity

In therapy, one of the therapist's core tasks is to understand the client, not only as an individual but also as someone shaped by early relationships and the broader sociocultural system in which they have developed. Societal systems, especially those that prioritise productivity, individualism and economic survival, leave limited space for connection and expression.

From the moment we are born, we rely on human contact and interaction for nurturing and development, and this is typically provided by parents or caregivers. However, these caregivers are themselves products of societal systems, which may not have served them well, depending on their many facets of identity.

In such cases, parents may struggle to engage with their new-borns or children from a non-verbal, emotional perspective, which we know is vital for human connection and development. Many of our interactions and experiences are unconsciously shaped by societal constructs and systems that we have normalised. These systems prioritise values like economic survival, often at the expense of emotional wellbeing. A glance at non-Western cultures reveals differing value systems; for instance, in some countries, shorter workdays allow more time for cultivating relationships, whether this is due to climate difference or cultural priorities, and this structure is beneficial for exploration of creativity and human connection.

Avery is a married, Christian, cisgendered, bisexual woman, of white British and Indian heritage. She is the mum of two young children, a four-year-old and a five-year-old. She has come to therapy with symptoms of exhaustion and, in her words, *an identity crisis*. She tries to balance her role as a parent with her personal life and work. She is overwhelmed with wanting to be a good-enough mother to her children, but struggles with the unrealistic expectations society has bestowed on her. She works a full-time 9–5 job with a one-hour commute to the office. The demands of her job means she often works past 5pm, getting home at 7pm most days. The family are barely making ends meet despite both parents working full-time jobs. They had to move away from their local area due to a rise in house prices.

Psychological impact on the family

- Avery has lost who she is and doesn't recognise herself in her role as a parent; she works long hours, which is leading to burnout and causing low mood.

- There is emotional distance between the parents and children as Avery returns home just before the children go to bed. The children lack play time with their parents because they are exhausted from working long hours. They are stretched to cover basic living requirements.

- This distance between the parents and children causes Avery to feel guilty, which negatively impacts her mood even further.

Advantages to the economic landscape and society

- Having two parents working full time means they are contributing to taxes, the economy and capitalism. These will help fund schools, healthcare, defence, etc.

Impact on identity

- Avery has stopped her usual hobbies. She loved to go to the gym but has stopped due to lack of time, money and energy. She has a keen interest in music and attending gigs, but has also stopped this, which has limited her social interactions.

- Avery is geographically further away from family and friends in a racially different area without people with similar backgrounds to her.

- Avery used to connect to her Indian roots by attending local community groups, but these are not present in her new area.

- Avery used to be active socially in her local LGBTQIA+ community, but this has changed since she moved house and she hasn't found a new group.

- Avery doesn't have time for hobbies or the downtime she had before children. She is socially isolated, feeling tired when she returns to the family home, and not having the emotional capacity to speak to friends. Her partner has a similar routine, although they are able to pick the children up from their after-school clubs.

- Avery doesn't have time to attend to her own self-care.

Western culture's emphasis on economic and technological advancement often sidelines emotional experiences. As Krause states: '...how the care-giver responds to a particular affect or behaviour in the infant will be contingent on the emotional acceptability of these displays to that care-giver within the care-giver's relational-cultural matrix' (2012, p.77). This highlights how relational and cultural contexts shape emotional responses and interactions from the earliest stages of life.

It would be naïve to think that capitalism does not contribute to the socioeconomic inequalities which have a direct effect on mental health services and resources. Disparities in income and employment can make it challenging for individuals to pay for private therapy. Although we are fortunate in the UK to have the NHS, we have seen the intense pressure it is currently under, with long waiting lists and staff exhaustion. In January 2025 the Royal College of Psychiatrists published an article which suggested that the number of people waiting to access mental health support had risen by 29 per cent in two years. Minutes from the House of Commons Women and Equalities Committee (2023) reported that there was a higher maternal mortality for Black and ethnically diverse women, with Black women almost four times more likely to die during childbirth. This highlights that there is a lack of cultural awareness among staff, which can affect someone's care, as well as the possibility of racial stereotypes, with this statistic showing that physical and mental health treatment vary depending on race, cultural background and identity.

This has gained more attention and publicity more recently, and although the government and the NHS report that they are wanting to reduce these rates, there has been little progress and improvement to date. The report from the Women and Equalities Committee (2023) discusses the socioeconomic factors that contribute to the health inequalities. MBRRACE-UK'S 2023 report stated there is a high link between the poorest and deprived areas and the highest mortality rates (MBRRACE-UK

2024). Moreover, it continues to explore that the greatest socioeconomic deprivation continues to affect ethnically minoritised people, thus influencing their mental health. Pressure is then placed on the individual to adjust their cultural attitudes, views and values to function in a society which oppresses them. People have had to change themselves to survive, and therapy has often helped people find ways to survive within these systems. Instead, what might be most beneficial would be to help improve a client's mental health while at the same time discouraging oppressive experiences and systems.

During the 1960s, we saw the Therapeutic Community Movement rise in the UK. Its main purpose was to offer the patient an environment in which they could participate in their therapeutic journey, as well as engage and form relationships with other patients and staff. Social factors were considered as an attempt to form treatment plans for the patient, and focused on how in-patients would interact and relate to one another (Tweedy 2017, p.21). Although the Therapeutic Community Movement is still being used or at least reflected on in many psychiatric settings to date, its popularity has seen a decrease due to the need to deconstruct institutionalisation. Mental health settings and in-patient wards were and are seen to be damaging to in-patients based on the view of isolation.

Even though the Therapeutic Community Movement attempts to include social interaction, it still places in-patients in confining spaces, and often treatments are impersonal, overlooking patients' identities and cultures. There is also a power imbalance and hierarchy within these systems that requires the in-patients to rely on mental health practitioners to help increase their wellbeing. Thus, more development in community work and housing patients within the community has more recently become a priority. The idea is to help individuals as they leave institutions, to continue their recovery in the outside world and among others, building on their emotional growth and becoming more independent because of this.

Bringing an awareness of systemic inequalities into therapy

Therapists need greater understanding of mental health and the overlapping of socioeconomic deprivation and systemic issues. With this understanding, we hope to enable a client to bring their authentic selves and experiences into therapy. As healthcare professionals, we need to start looking differently into a person's experience. We must begin to look at people through their unique circumstances. For example, therapists are often called to work with children and adolescents demonstrating 'low self-esteem', 'behavioural issues' and lower achievement levels within the school environment. The onus is primarily placed on the young person to change. For many young people, if they are unable to integrate into school systems, they are met with repercussions, such as exclusion or detentions. This can exacerbate their isolation, making them feel further isolated and 'othered'. They are met with labels such as 'interruptive', 'aggressive' or 'underachieving' by professionals and educators. The lack of curiosity from therapists as to what is causing the young person to struggle in the school environment is where systems fail them. (Unless therapists are systemically trained to look into systems, this will hinder their curiosity.)

Growing up in poverty is stressful for both adults and children. There is no escaping the fact that living conditions vary and are often compromised. Space can be limited in working-class homes. Some families may share bedrooms, meaning there is limited private space to unwind or reset. Walls within terraced homes or flats are often thinner, and subsequent noise levels can influence an individual's ability to concentrate, making tasks such as homework harder to manage and complete. Moreover, there is less food and resources within financially insecure homes. All these factors significantly influence someone's physical and mental wellbeing.

Before starting therapy, a therapist should assess the systemic issues affecting a client to determine if they are ready for therapy. Considering and addressing the following factors can help a therapist or practitioner decide how to approach the therapeutic process to best meet a client's needs:

- Are the client's living conditions stable enough for them to participate in a therapeutic intervention? Stability will help with engagement with therapy and figuring out what they are wanting out of a therapy or therapeutic intervention. This may involve collaboration with other services to help establish a safe and stable environment for the client – whether this is within your own organisation, private practice or other agency.

- Does the client have a good support system around them, and can they identify a trusted person or people? This could include other professionals and individuals a client can call on to help in times of struggle. It can help to prevent dependency on therapy or therapeutic intervention.

- Are you working to co-produce a suitable therapeutic plan with the client? In this process, the client and therapist work together, with the therapist inviting the client to share their experiences relating to their socioeconomic background and other elements of their identity.

- Does the client need individual therapeutic support or community care? Is there pressure for an individualistic approach to the therapeutic intervention, due to systemic factors?

- How can therapy help challenge the status quo, capitalism and oppressive systems instead of turning mental health into another productivity machine?

- Are you looking at the client via a holistic lens and providing a space to explore and promote justice and equality?

Working cross-culturally in therapy

Focusing on identity and cultural work in therapy creates strong foundations for positive and healthy relationships within therapy and our communities. In recent decades, dominant cultural models within therapy have influenced how we interact and what we choose to exhibit in front of others. Practitioners and clients should be encouraged to develop a balanced approach of working together, where they can bring in their cultural knowledge to reconnect them with their cultural experiences while simultaneously strengthening their identity. This process gives clients autonomy and develops their expertise in making sense of their narratives.

What does cross-cultural therapy involve?

Remaining open-minded and respectful when working with clients is vital during cross-cultural therapeutic work. It involves collaborating and engaging with others who may not form part of your own cultural background or beliefs and working with the difference. Providing culturally appropriate therapeutic interventions is at the centre of the work. These interventions enable clients to navigate through their own culture within therapy, while the therapist also remains culturally present within their own cultural identity.

Working cross-culturally invites collaboration between the client and therapist to bridge cultural difference via a therapeutic intervention, and makes room for effective communication. Difference can feel uncomfortable to engage in, and this discomfort can provoke a desire to avoid this challenging area of therapeutic work and move into the familiarity of sameness. Effective and sensitive communication is important, as communication can vary cross-culturally. For example, clients may seek therapy knowing little or no English, and their inability to communicate in the most widely spoken language in the UK may have contributed to a sense of isolation within their communities and social surroundings. If our client's cultural experiences do not match the culture around them, they may feel socially excluded and forced to adapt and conform on a day-to-day basis.

Therapists should be mindful of a client's difference, even if it is not being verbally communicated. Non-verbal communication, such as body language, visual cues and gestures, may indicate a client's cultural values, cultural customs and beliefs. Taking a culturally sensitive approach is important when developing and delivering therapeutic interventions.

> **Aisha is a 34-year-old woman** from the Muslim community. Aisha is attending her first session with a new therapist who is male. The therapist notices that Aisha does not engage in extended eye contact with him. He is mindful of cultural differences and realises that Aisha's limited eye contact may relate to Islamic beliefs and customs about interaction with people of the opposite gender. To show that he acknowledges and respects Aisha's cultural differences, the therapist adapts his own eye contact accordingly. He also asks Aisha

direct questions about her needs and wants from therapy, including whether she would prefer to work with a therapist of the same gender. Aisha says that she would feel more comfortable speaking to a female therapist, so he proposes re-referring her to a suitable therapist.

Responsive cross-cultural therapy

Cultural differences often show up in subtle ways. For example, some cultures use their body to communicate certain feelings more than they use words. In other cultures, the tone of voice that is used to share a story or experience can be significant. This can be the case in the Cypriot community. Cypriots are known for using body language and hand gestures to emphasise their points, and for often speaking at a high volume and a fast pace. These verbal and non-verbal behaviours are used to vividly convey the points that they are trying to communicate. However, these cultural differences have often been misinterpreted as aggression. It is important for therapists to sensitively interpret such differences and avoid passing judgement.

Of course, not all Cypriots will use expressive body language and nor will all Muslim clients limit eye contact with someone of the opposite gender in therapy. Despite this, it can greatly benefit the therapeutic relationship if therapists undertake their own research into their clients' cultures and cultural experiences of the world. Research and understanding enables therapists to develop their cultural knowledge and to notice certain verbal or non-verbal cues that a client brings into the therapeutic space. We can, if appropriate, bring these cues into the consciousness of the therapeutic relationship.

Prompts to support effective cross-cultural practice

These phrases may empower clients to bring their culture and identity into the therapeutic room:

> I can see how much this means to you and how important it is for me to understand...

I have noticed you using your body to communicate certain feelings and stories with me.

What do you need from therapy in order for you to bring your whole self into this space?

Is there anything I can do to help facilitate a space where you can bring your identity and culture into the space?

Bringing an awareness of cross-cultural differences into therapy

Therapy can be a cultural shock for many clients. Due to this, clients may feel the need to significantly adapt their individual experiences with culture to adjust to the therapeutic environment. Clients will come to therapy with multiple identities, such as sexuality, gender, race, heritage and class. The pressure to integrate into society can diminish these aspects of identity, but therapy can strengthen clients' cultural connections. A willingness to learn from clients and develop an understanding of their cultural backgrounds is core to effective cross-cultural therapy.

Understanding protected characteristics in therapy

In the UK, some aspects of identity are legally protected from discrimination. Familiarity with these 'protected characteristics' provides a helpful platform from which therapists can explore other intersections. This foundational knowledge will support you to use the activities in Part 2 with sensitivity and understanding.

We will give you examples to illustrate how parts of our identity intersect with more familiar ones. When we say 'protected characteristics', we refer to those as listed by the UK government. We are using this as a frame to give you background to discussing other intersections. It is tempting to list every single identity here and go through them one by one, but we would like to use each characteristic and integrate them in order to consider identity in a holistic way:

- Age
- Race, including colour, nationality, ethnic or national origin
- Religion or belief
- Gender reassignment, sex, sexual orientation
- Being married or in a civil partnership, being pregnant or on maternity leave.

Protected characteristics are important in therapy because it means people are safeguarded by the Equality Act 2010, protecting people from discrimination. This is a legal framework that can support clients as well as therapists if they feel discriminated against within and outside the therapy room.

Working with neurodiversity in therapy

Neurodiversity describes the natural differences in human brains. Neurodivergent people's brains work differently to those of neurotypical people, and this affects their experiences of the world. Neurodivergent conditions include autism, ADHD, dyslexia and dyspraxia.

The neurodiversity movement, which embraces multiple forms of neurological diversity, was developed to challenge the ways in which people view and marginalise autistic people. Early narratives around neurodiversity often led to the pathologising of autistic individuals, framing them as a burden. In her book *Autism Is Not a Disease: The Politics of Neurodiversity*, Jodie Hare examines how the medical model has contributed to this harmful perspective. She highlights Nick Walker's pathology paradigm, which is rooted in two key assumptions: first, that there is a single 'right' and 'healthy' way for human brains to function, and second, that any deviation from this dominant mode of thinking or being is inherently 'unhealthy' or indicative of something 'wrong' (Hare 2024, p.18).

Working with neurodiverse clients in therapy

Therapeutic sessions may need to be adapted to best meet clients' needs. When working with a neurodivergent client, it is paramount that we educate ourselves around their specific form of neurodivergence. Not all clients who are neurodivergent will require the same interventions. Every neurodivergent person is different and experiences and interacts with the world in a distinct way. For example, an autistic client may be sensory sensitive. A client with ADHD may face challenges with executive functioning, such as setting goals or managing tasks. As with all our clients, we must centre a client's specific needs when we are making formulations and clinical decisions in therapy. A therapist should focus on the client's strengths within sessions rather than pathologising their differences.

Leon is a 24-year-old autistic man who has decided to refer himself to therapy to help him manage his anxiety and sensory overwhelm at work. Leon has chosen to work with Maya, an art psychotherapist. Leon has chosen art psychotherapy partly because he struggles to verbally articulate his feelings, and he dislikes long periods of eye contact.

First session

During the first session Leon has an open conversation with Maya, informing her that a 50-minute session may not be ideal for him due to sensory overwhelm. Maya leads with curiosity and wants to know what else may benefit Leon during their sessions. Leon explains that he is sensitive to noise and bright lights.

Therapeutic space adaptation

Maya considers Leon's needs in order for therapy to be more accessible for him and his needs. Maya ensures that the lights are dimmed before Leon's sessions, that there are clay and fidget toys in the therapeutic room for Leon to use should he need to self-regulate and ground himself. She also provides headphones to help with any loud noises during creative activities. Leon's session is shortened to 35 minutes.

Benefits of therapeutic adaptation

After several weeks of Leon engaging in art psychotherapy with Maya, he feels comfortable with the routine and the therapeutic space and its adaptations. As therapy progresses Leon realises that his ability to stay engaged within the session has strengthened, and this is partly to do with this flexibility that was communicated and created between him and his therapist.

The traditional form of psychotherapy, a 50-minute session, may not be optimal when working with a neurodivergent client. This could be due to a client being unable to remain focused or sit still for that duration of time. In such instances a shorter session may decrease overwhelm. In contrast, a neurodivergent client who processes information slowly may benefit from a longer session. Therapists may also need to adapt their space to best meet different clients' specific needs. Involving clients in therapeutic planning will help to establish the best intervention for them.

Prompts for working effectively with neurodivergent clients

- How does your client's neurodivergence define and affect them? What does neurodiversity mean to them? Do dominant cultures and systems bypass their needs?
- Can anything within the therapeutic environment be adjusted to meet your client's needs?
- How does the client like to communicate? Do they have non-verbal ways of communicating?
- Could the duration of sessions be adapted to decrease anxiety around the length of time of therapy?
- Have you involved the client, or (where appropriate) parent or caregiver, in the planning of therapy? Inviting clients to participate in their own therapeutic planning centres the client and their needs.
- Does your client experience sensitivity to noise? If they do, they may want to wear headphones within the session to increase concentration and ground them. Formulate a plan with the client around this.

- Could it be beneficial to use sensory objects during therapy? Sensory objects can be incorporated into sessions to provide comfort. For example, a client may need something tactile or comforting, such as a blanket.

- Have you noticed any visible changes in a client's presentation during therapy? If so, have you reflected on what these changes may mean? For example, if a client is fidgeting more frequently than usual, it might indicate that they feel overwhelmed.

- What do you think the silences in your sessions mean to your client? How do you think they feel during periods of silence? Silences in therapy can feel different for neurodivergent clients.

Bringing an awareness of neurodivergence into therapy

It is important to remember that not all difference is visible when working with neurodivergent clients. Therapists should take a flexible approach and avoid rigid therapeutic frameworks. This will enable nuanced practice that recognises and embraces clients' individual needs. By increasing our awareness of clients' needs and working collaboratively, therapists can support clients to find therapeutic interventions that work for them. Therapists can do this by creatively adapting therapeutic sessions to accommodate their clients, making therapy accessible and bringing clients' voices into therapeutic planning.

Working with gender, sexuality and relationship status in therapy

Gender, sexuality and relationship status are aspects of identity that hold significant importance within Western culture, particularly in the 21st century. From birth, individuals are placed within the male and female gender binary. As we progress through life, we encounter various forms with questions that require us to define ourselves in terms of these parts of our identity. The complexity of gender, sexuality and relationship status is often diminished by the use of simplistic binaries: gender as male or female; sexuality as heterosexual or homosexual; and relationship status as either single or in a monogamous relationship.

Moving beyond binary frameworks

For those who do not conform to these cultural norms, navigating these layers of identity can be challenging. Additionally, many individuals in the UK may come from families with generational ties to other countries, meaning they often navigate multiple cultural perspectives on these issues. This highlights the importance of exploring these topics with clients to better understand how dominant cultural views shape their experiences and challenges.

A client's difficulties are often rooted in the constraints imposed by dominant cultural narratives. Therefore, it is essential to move beyond binary frameworks and to develop a deeper understanding of the assumptions and projections that arise from them. By doing so, therapists can better support clients in navigating and challenging these cultural norms.

Developing gender awareness in therapy

Gender can be an important part of your client's cultural identity. This can be seen or unseen, voiced or unvoiced. Being culturally competent using gender as a lens is not a case of only asking a person's pronouns. We are all judged on how we present ourselves to the world and the body we show each other (Hogan 2019). Mental health challenges and diagnoses have typically been a gendered experience. Women are more likely to receive a diagnosis of borderline personality disorder compared to men, who are more likely to receive a diagnosis of anti-social personality disorder. We must hold this in mind when faced with clients with specific diagnoses. In recent years, there has been a cultural shift in that more women are receiving a diagnosis of ADHD and autism, whereas historically more men received these diagnoses. The Royal College of Psychiatrists states the male-female 'sex ratio has narrowed from 9:1 to closer to 2:1' for an autism diagnosis (2024).

Referrals for gender exploration within clinical services in the UK have risen in recent years. One study found that 'the rate of transgender identity recorded in primary care records has increased fivefold from 2000 to 2018 and is highest in the 16–17 and 18–29 age groups' (McKechnie, D.G.J. *et al.* 2023, p.1). Adult services have followed a similar trend over recent times: 'waiting lists have increased by 20,698 (144%)...over the last five years' (Prosho 2024, p.25). Exploring a person's gender identity may be a 'new' part of identity that experienced therapists may be unfamiliar working within. It is therefore extremely important that you do not assume that clients have a 'problem' with their gender if this differs from their gender assigned at birth. The activities in this book are designed to inform and enrich your work with all clients, regardless of the way they initially present their gender. While it may be tempting to focus on these activities when working with a transgender client, it's important to keep intersectionality in mind and consider gender as an important facet of every client's identity.

Reflect on what it means to be your gender, or how your relationship with your gender has changed over time. Like all the other aspects of intersectionality, gender does not exist on its own: we must consider it within the context of factors such as religion, environment, race, culture and socioeconomic background. This goes for the client and us as therapists or practitioners. For example, if a person of colour comes to therapy who is non-binary and wanting to explore gender and race, but we avoid addressing the added structural inequality of race, it can lead to inadequate support. People's lived experiences are a product of their intersections, and recognising all intersections of identity is important, as this will give us an overview of where social systems fail different parts of our clients' intersections.

> **Priti is a 35-year-old Muslim** client born to immigrant parents. She struggles with her sense of self and feels uncomfortable with male attention. Her therapist introduces an activity that explores gender within therapy and provides space for Priti to decide whether she would like to engage in it. Allowing Priti to use her own agency and offering her a choice validates Priti's experiences. Priti was left feeling seen and heard by her therapist.

Sophia, a heterosexual female client with low mood who struggles with romantic relationships, attends therapy seeking to create a better understanding of herself. Sophia's therapist introduces her to a gender activity in a way to explore her relationship with herself and the male gaze. During the activity Sophia and her therapist reflect on how she presents her female self in relation to her culture, religion, spiritual self and the environment she was raised in. During her engagement with the activity she reflects on: How does her presentation affect how others relate to her, others in her family, work and social life? Is she able to reflect on her femininity and/or sexuality throughout her life up until now?

Prompts for exploring gender in therapy with clients

- Could your own biases negatively affect your client's healing? If so, consider a different therapist while you actively work on addressing these biases.

- Are your competencies strong enough in this area? Your lack of work on exploring your own gender, sexuality and relationships could negatively affect your client in ways that are not visible to you.

- How does your client feel in your presence? When working on gender with your client, check in on how they feel – this may be verbally or non-verbally. Not everyone will be able to say they are uncomfortable, and some clients may be hesitant to express themselves in front of their therapist. Are you of a different gender to your client? If so, this may influence how they express themselves in your presence. A client's perceptions of your religion, age, sexuality and other aspects of identity may also affect your therapeutic relationship.

- Are you using language sensitively? Be mindful of the language you use with clients, as biases can easily creep into the language we use, even if we believe that we are being inclusive. For example, you may speak to a female client about motherhood and having children when you may not speak to a male client in this way.

- Are you taking a cross-cultural approach to exploring gender? The majority of current therapeutic teachings are rooted in white Western teachings. This has an impact on how we approach conversations around gender, sexuality and relationship status. Understanding a client's heritage and other dominant cultures through the lens of gender, sexuality and relationship status is important.

- How do you present your gender at work? Does this change, and why? Consider how you present your gender and how you feel in your body when at work or while working with specific clients; this often changes depending on who you work with.

Gender is a facet of someone's identity, and it does not completely define them. Therapists need to think about a person as a whole and how aspects of their identity intersect. It is important to avoid making assumptions about a person's relationship with their gender or their gender expression. Exploring our own prejudices and judgements, and how these have been shaped by our own cultural upbringing, is essential when providing treatment for a person who wishes to explore this part of their identity.

Developing an awareness of sexuality in therapy

The expression of sexuality is a core part of a person's identity, and it is therefore an important identity-based characteristic to explore in therapy. A client's ability and freedom to express their sexuality and gender will be influenced by many factors, including their environment, the law, their class, religion, gender and job.

People from the LGBTQIA+ community face significantly more barriers to mental health support than cisgendered heterosexual people. This is widely discussed in professional spaces, but how might other aspects of identity relating to someone's community or background affect their access to support? For example, an African, Muslim, queer man may navigate further cultural and religious barriers to seeking help. If a therapist has conflicting beliefs about a person's sexuality, this can lead to a negative and potentially traumatic therapeutic experience.

Jo, a queer, non-binary young adult, started therapy with a cisgendered female therapist with limited knowledge of gender and sexual expression. The therapist has not asked Jo for their pronouns.

Jo initially referred themselves to therapy to explore multiple aspects of their identity with their therapist. Jo has been struggling with communicating their sexuality and gender with peers and family, which is causing them sleepless nights and anxiety.

Challenge

Jo has sought therapy to explore multiple aspects of their identity, including sexuality and gender. From the outset Jo began to feel unsafe in the therapeutic relationship, where pronouns were not acknowledged or thought about. This lack of attunement increased the risk of misgendering, reinforcing the client's sense of invisibility. The therapist, although well-meaning, was unaware of the potential harm caused by not actively creating an affirming space for gender-diverse clients.

During one session

At one point, the therapist introduced a creative exercise around sexuality, assuming this would be helpful due to the client's perceived queer identity. However, the intervention felt premature and disconnected from where the client was in their processing. The client has not yet disclosed or processed their feelings about gender and felt the activity placed pressure on them to label or perform an identity they were still exploring privately.

Prompts for exploring sexuality in therapy

When exploring sexuality through creative work in therapeutic practice, the following reflective prompts can help deepen awareness and dialogue:

- What creative images, colours, movements or materials help you express or explore aspects of your sexual identity?
- Are there parts of your sexuality that feel easier to express non-verbally than through words?
- How have societal or cultural messages influenced the way you experience and embody your sexuality?
- In what ways can creativity help you reconnect with pleasure, desire or shame in a safe and held space?
- What might it feel like to co-create something with another person that reflects your lived experience of sexuality?

Developing an awareness of relationship status in therapy

A client's relationship status, whether single, married, divorced, widowed, polyamorous or monogamous, or in any other non-traditional or non-conventional dynamic, will play a significant part in a client's identity and their experiences within the world around them. Relationships affect many other parts of our identity intersections, such as religion and culture, for example. They can affect our emotional wellbeing and self-concept.

Therapists should explore the following with their clients:

- How do you define your relationship(s) status? What does this mean to you?

- Are there any cultural or societal pressures and differences you have experienced due to your relationship(s) status?
- Have there been any barriers you have experienced within these relationships?

TOM IS A 52-YEAR-OLD, CISGENDERED, CHRISTIAN WHITE MAN

He had been married to his wife of 28 years who sadly passed away three years ago. Tom feels the grief of his significant loss. He also feels lost in his new identity as a single, widowed man and is struggling to adapt to this way of living. He shows signs of low mood and loneliness. Tom has reached out for therapy because he is keen to find another partner but is nervous to start dating again after being in a marriage for so long to his first girlfriend.

Therapy

Tom's therapist initially focuses on grief and loss in Tom's world; however, it becomes apparent that he is struggling with his new identity as a single man. He is cautious to 'start again'. It becomes clear that Tom has been impacted by wider society's image of a single man in his 50s and how his peers and family ask him if he has found anyone yet. This makes him feel isolated. Therapy helps Tom to recognise his low mood in the societal context of being single as a middle-aged man. Therapy also helps Tom to connect how his faith impacts his feelings around dating again.

Understanding ability and disability in therapeutic spaces

There are many definitions of disability, but in this book we use the definition given by GOV.UK under the Equality Act 2010: a 'physical or mental impairment that has a "substantial" and "long-term" negative effect on your ability to do normal daily activities'.[1] Disabilities can be seen or unseen, and when you are working with a client you cannot make assumptions about their ability based on how they present. For example, if

1 www.gov.uk/definition-of-disability-under-equality-act-2010

a person uses a mobility aid, this may be an obvious visual cue suggesting that they have a physical disability. However, some mental health conditions are unseen disabilities that you may not register in the therapeutic space unless you ask clients relevant questions.

When exploring identity, it is important to be mindful of how clients with disabilities are perceived in wider society. In the UK, evidence suggests that disability dominates other aspects of people's intersectional identities. For example, people with a disability may not be asked about relationships, sex and intimacy (Halacre 2021). Disability as an identity can be overlooked or bring unwanted attention. Mary Wickenden (2023) states that when someone is labelled as disabled their other intersections are erased and their disability takes focus, drawing attention away from other aspects of identity.

The wider representation of disabled people can also be problematic. Halacre (2021) describes how disabled people are not represented in pop culture and are often stereotyped as white, straight and middle class; this limits their visibility as people with many intersections. Such cultural representations may influence able-bodied clinicians to unknowingly reinforce these stereotypes. We must practise reflexivity and be conscious of our own biases and assumptions when working with disabled clients. It is important that we do not judge a disabled person by one intersection of their identity but recognise their complexity and individuality. As everyone has multiple identities and identity ebbs, flows and shifts, your client with a disability may or may not see their disability as part of their identity.

Melanie, a 28-year-old woman with a physical disability diagnosed in early childhood, was referred to therapy with a desire to explore feelings of isolation and low self-esteem. She reported difficulty forming romantic relationships and uncertainty about her role in society as a disabled adult woman.

Melanie's therapy sessions explore her intersectional identity. The therapist and Melanie look at how her gender and disability interact with each other and how this has formed Melanie's experiences with relationships and sexuality.

Melanie opens up to her therapist and shares that she has encountered both ableist attitudes and gendered expectations from people in society. She gives examples of people seeing her as asexual or dependent, which she explains have had an effect on her confidence, asserting her needs and desires in relationships.

Therapy sessions

Therapy with Melanie focused on:

- Building a safe and trusting therapeutic relationship to allow space for exploring sensitive topics.
- Validating Melanie's lived experiences of exclusion and misunderstanding.
- Exploring barriers Melanie faced in adolescence around developing autonomy and identity.
- Encouraging dialogue around self-worth, sexuality and aspirations that challenge both internalised and societal limitations.

The British Association for Counselling and Psychotherapy (BACP) guidance on working with disability (Halacre 2021) shares how some clients may not have been able to access the same opportunities during adolescence to explore risk-taking boundaries, sexuality and independence. If you are working with a disabled client, it is important to explore parts of their intersectionality while learning what barriers they may have encountered growing up or since acquiring their disability. As with other aspects of identity you must have a working relationship with your client which feels safe before discussing sensitive topics.

Wickenden (2023) goes on to link the disadvantages disabled women in particular experience, relating gender to ability. Women with disabilities experience challenges due to the way their bodies are viewed when thinking of traditional gender norms such as domesticity, having children and being wives. They have to navigate ableist societal structures in order to reach services.

Removing barriers to therapy

Disabled clients may experience practical barriers that could inhibit access to therapy, such as needing physical assistance, interpreters or personal assistants. In therapy spaces, access mobility may not be set up for a disabled client. The duration of the session may need to be adapted to suit their needs. A client may experience fatigue from the additional factors needed to set up a therapeutic intervention (Halacre 2021). Halacre describes the emotional labour that can be caused by medication, pain or sleep, for example. It is important to be mindful that disabled clients may need to do a lot of practical preparation in order to attend therapy.

Prompts for engaging with ability and disability in therapy

The following prompts are given here as guidance to use with clients when engaging and exploring ability and disability within the therapeutic setting:

- How do you identify in terms of ability and disability, and what does this mean to you?
- How does your experience with disability intersect with other aspects of your identity, such as relationships, work, gender, etc....?
- Has there ever been a time you have felt seen or unseen due to your disability, and what was this experience like for you?
- What messages did you receive in terms of disability from family, friends and social settings?
- Are there assumptions people have made about you, your body and your ability that has impacted you?
- Shall we explore your own needs, desires and the emotional and physical boundaries which may impact them?

As therapists, we must learn and understand the barriers that people with disabilities face in order to make adaptations and create positive therapeutic relationships. These suggestions can support you to work effectively with disabled clients:

- How might your identity influence the therapeutic relationship? For example, Wickenden (2023) states that '[disabled] women may not feel welcomed in women's conversations or events', reinforcing their feelings of otherness and isolation. If a disabled woman is seeking therapeutic support from a female therapist, how will this play out in therapy if left unspoken? Acknowledging and exploring the relationship between client and practitioner is key as a foundation to change.

- What do the intersections of their identity mean to your client? If you are working with a disabled client, it can be useful to go through the intersectionality diagram from Chapter 1 to focus on the different intersections of connections between parts of their identity.

- Have you made assumptions about your client's identity? Considering intersectionality can be confusing if a person may not relate their ability or disability to their identity and vice versa. We must treat each person as unique in how they view identity, and not make assumptions towards their experience. This is a tentative balancing act as you may feel it is important to explore this part of their presentation.

EXPLORING ASSUMPTIONS

As we have learned, ability and disability can be negatively isolated into a singular intersection. We must attempt to unlearn this unhelpful perception to avoid bringing it into the therapeutic space. This activity can help us to break down our own judgements on ability and disability, and to view the abilities of ourselves and our clients differently.

- Step 1: Pick a client or focus on yourself.
- Step 2: List the 'social graces' (see Chapter 1) and consider how ability and disability may affect each intersection and how you imagine this to be so. Jot this down on a piece of paper.
- Step 3: Did you notice anything you missed at first? Did you realise any assumptions or biases?

As with all aspects of identity, exploring ability and disability is complex and variable. To build trusting therapeutic relationships with disabled clients, you must work responsively and flexibly at the client's pace.

Working with religion and spirituality in therapy

Religion is an important aspect of many people's identities in the UK. According to the 2021 Census in England and Wales, 46.2 per cent of people identified as Christian, 37.2 per cent as no religion, 6.5 per cent as Muslim, 1.7 per cent as Hindu, 0.9 per cent as Sikh, 0.5 per cent as Jewish and 0.6 per cent described themselves as 'Other'. Culturally, many people across the UK follow Christian traditions and follow a Christian calendar. Some school holidays are scheduled around Christian events such as Easter and Christmas, and many people celebrate festivals that are rooted in Christianity. The integration of the Christian calendar into UK societal celebrations and public holidays illustrates religious privilege and highlights how dominant cultural systems influence public norms and traditions.

For some people, religion gives them strength that guides them through life and brings comfort in times of despair. When it comes to therapy, bringing in a client's religious beliefs may add value to interventions and their overall outcomes, but this may be dependent on the therapist's own religious or spiritual beliefs.

Differences in religious beliefs can impact the approach the therapist takes. If a client's religion remains unvoiced and unseen, this may mean that the client's religious identity is not explored in therapy, even though it is important to them.

> **STEPHEN IS A 38-YEAR-OLD MAN.** He has recently started private therapy. Stephen travels weekly to his therapist's home where therapy takes place. Stephen is spiritual and religious. He regularly attends church – it is where he gets community support and where he reads scripture, which acts as a form of guidance during difficult times. Stephen hasn't noticed any signs in the therapeutic space that suggest that his therapist might be religious or spiritual. This has made Stephen apprehensive to share his religion with his therapist, out of fear of being judged or dismissed.

The therapist's identity and perspective

The therapist is a female psychotherapist who is an atheist. She believes in working with whatever the client brings to the session. She is committed to remaining neutral in therapy, and does not believe in bringing her own beliefs or worldviews into the therapeutic space.

Missed opportunities

- Stephen's religion remains unseen and unvoiced; therefore, the therapist misses a significant aspect of Stephen's identity which provides him with coping mechanisms.

- If the therapist was aware of this, religion and spirituality could be included in Stephen's care plans and intervention.

- Stephen is unable to bring his full authentic self into therapy out of fear of being judged or misunderstood. Therefore, Stephen's progress in therapy is slower as he is censoring aspects of his identity.

- Stephen's community support through his church is not explored in therapy, which could be included in his care plans and therapeutic interventions.

Prompts for exploring religion and spirituality during therapy

- Is religion and spirituality an important part of your identity?
- Would you like to include aspects of your religious and spiritual practice in our work together?
- Are there any spiritual or religious customs or rituals that you feel I [as the therapist] should be aware of in supporting you?

- Are there any times in which you may be observing a religious festival that we may need to work around in therapy?
- Would you feel comfortable sharing more with me about your religion and spirituality and worldview?

Therapeutic interventions must make space for the client to bring any element of their identity into a session. Creativity creates a powerful pathway for this exploration, allowing clients to express themselves beyond words to bring to consciousness parts of their identity that may have otherwise been silenced and overlooked. This not only enriches the therapeutic journey for the client, but it also affirms their humanity.

PART 2

Creative Activities

In this part of the book we focus on creative activities from a variety of professionals who use creativity to explore identity and culture. Contributors have shared their own identity using a particular cultural lens as a focus. Furthermore, the activities offer a systematic guide on how to use creativity in a session with a client, and to further explore identity and culture within the therapeutic experience. These activities are flexible. They can be completed with a client within one-to-one therapy, group therapy or even supervision. The therapist or practitioner and client can adapt the activities as they wish, taking into account the client's needs. Activities can be completed together with the client and/or the client can complete the activity alone outside of the therapy room. Moreover, an activity can be used as a conversation. The client may not wish to engage with creative material as such, but may want to explore the activity verbally.

There is no specific order to these activities – they should be thought of as 'ingredients' and not 'recipes', meaning we can tweak or change them as we go along, making them more individual and catered to our clients. We would caveat that the client should be placed at the centre of their identity and culture exploration work. We are not the experts of our client's journey, and there needs to be a collective approach with the creative engagement.

For ease of reading, the activities have been grouped into five chapters, covering body exploration (Chapter 3), words and movement (Chapter 4), geography, music and food (Chapter 5), safety (Chapter 6) and reflection (Chapter 7). These are only loose themes, and some of the activities may cross over.

Please encourage your client (and yourself) to take breaks in between activities. Activities can feel heavy, so notice how you are feeling within your body, give space for your client to simultaneously notice, and respond to this. Ask your client to take a moment out after each activity and to focus on what may be happening within their own bodies. Identity and culture exploration can hold a lot of shame and trauma, which may not be directly linked to the client themselves, but have been passed down through generations and through normative social systems.

We encourage these activities to be used when an established, 'safe enough' and 'good enough' environment (Winnicott 1971) between the therapist and client has been formed. A client must feel emotional safety and physical safety, in order to make room for creativity and play. These activities should help foster creativity and emotional wellbeing. By helping our clients work through their multiple layers of identity and emotions, we hope that they can begin to develop a sense of self, autonomy and agency within their communities and cultures.

It is also important to note that some of these activities may read longer than others. We have had contributions from creative therapists and individuals who have shared parts of their own identity within their creative contributions to this book, so please take your time to read through their introduction and narrative, which may help explain their creative contribution further.

Overall, we hope that these activities can help you, your clients and colleagues gain a deeper understanding of themselves and the world around them: '...the act of creation is an attempt to enter a mysterious realm, a longing to transcend. What we create allows us to share glimpses of an inner landscape, one that is beyond our understanding. Art is our portal to the unseen world' (Rubin 2023, p.31).

The effect of creation is difficult to describe using words, but Rubin puts it nicely here, as a way of sharing one's inner world with another person. This is what we are asking our clients to do when using these activities. We are asking them to go into a realm of the unknown, to activate their spiritual selves, and to share the unknown with their therapist.

CHAPTER 3

Exploring Culture and Identity through Body Exploration

Map of you

Tia Terefe, art psychotherapist and Internal Family Systems therapist

Have you ever wondered about what makes you, you, why you are drawn to certain hobbies or areas of interest, why you tend to act a certain way? Or what influenced your preference of area to live in? Maybe you have wondered about how other people perceive you or how you feel when someone else describes you? I know I have spent time wondering about these questions myself at various stages in my life.

I was born a triplet in Ethiopia, separated at birth from my mother and siblings, and later adopted in Sweden at two-and-a-half months old. The rural community I grew up in was all-white. There was no one who understood my skin care needs or how to care for my afro hair. No one to help me maintain links with or teach me about my Ethiopian heritage. The world around me was 'white' and this was all I knew for many years.

I later left home at the age of 18 with the aim of finding a place where I could 'blend in' and to find people I could identify with. City life was both exciting and challenging as I learned to manage life without the safety net I had known being part of a family unit with white parents. I looked like a young Ethiopian woman, but my worldview, language, identity and name were 'white' and culturally Swedish. This caused issues and confusion when attending job interviews, moving to new neighbourhoods, travelling, and so on.

At the age of 20, I connected with others who had also been adopted from Ethiopia to Sweden. Some of us had never known or met other adoptees before and we felt deeply connected by our shared experiences. We could express ourselves fully without being told that we were 'lucky to be adopted', that we were 'ungrateful' for wanting to search for our biological families, or judged because we didn't speak Amharic.

Transracial or transnational adoptees and clients who have lived in foster care or guardianship with carers of a different 'race' may have additional layers of loss and complex life experiences. Therapists who welcome these clients into their space need to learn about concepts of white privilege, white supremacy, racism, microaggression, internalised racism, racial identity formation and the impact of complex trauma. Therapists can support clients by learning about these and other relevant issues to avoid doing the work 'colour blind'.

'All parts are welcome' is an Internal Family Systems therapy phrase that I hold dear. This method of working opens a safe and compassionate dialogue with the parts of ourselves we may normally suppress or battle with. Learning to identify, listen to and allow for these parts to be seen and heard can bring about significant change and a stronger sense of Self. I invite you to pause here, to take a breath and notice what comes up for you as you read this activity. Any thoughts or feelings around transracial adoption, community, identity, white privilege, racism, working with clients of another 'race'? Maybe you noticed something that surprised you or was uncomfortable to feel? See if you can gently allow for all parts to be acknowledged as they show up. You can write them down or use art materials to draw anything you find important to perhaps follow up on. If it feels right for you, take a moment to thank the parts for letting you know what was shared before moving your focus elsewhere. This brief check-in can be used to better understand your thoughts and feelings around working with the activity explained next.

MAP OF YOU (55 MINUTES)

Aim: To explore identity and intersectionality.

What you will need: The sheet of paper with prompts (see below) (these can be cut out and laminated or used as a whole table of prompts), white paper for drawing (no smaller than A3) and crayons or felt tip pens.

Introduce the activity (10 minutes): This activity invites you to explore identity and intersectionality with your clients in a creative way. It can easily be adapted to fit different age groups by changing the words or by using appropriate images. It can be used within a single session to map out the basics or be explored during several sessions by focusing in-depth on different areas within the initial map.

Draw an outline of a body on the white paper (5 minutes).

Present the prompts and invite the client to choose what prompts to start with (20 minutes, drawing and writing):

- Ask the client to focus on one prompt at a time.
- Invite the client to notice any sensations they may feel in their own body as they do this.
- Ask them to pay attention to any other responses they may have (an image, memory, symbol, colour, etc.).
- Invite the client to draw the image/symbol/colour on the white paper. They can draw within or outside the outline of the body.

Add a few words next to each drawing to help identify each response.

Reflections and questions for the client (15 minutes)

- What identities are most important to you?
- What identities do you find easy/difficult to relate to?
- What parts hold power and/or privilege?
- How do you feel towards your response to each prompt?
- Do you feel curious to learn more about any of the identities? If so, why?
- Are you aware of what values are praised/what beliefs would be challenging to disagree with? If yes, explain what these are.
- What are your thoughts or feelings around what role race/age/gender had within the family or community you grew up in? What, if anything, has changed?
- How is mental health/sexual orientation/religion understood in your culture or family?
- Who is an important role model within your family or community?
- Who in your family or community racially mirrors you?
- What identities seem to highlight how others perceive you?
- Is there anything you would change if you could go back in time?
- Is there anything you would like to change looking ahead?
- What thoughts, feelings or physical responses do you have as you look at the finished drawing?
- What did you learn that was new about yourself or the world around you?

Ending (5 minutes): Once you've completed the activity, take a moment to look at your creation. Notice whether any parts of your identity feel like they need more attention. You might find something that surprised you or highlighted an area of growth. Allow whatever comes up to be there.

Please use the following prompts, and you can also add your own. This page is available to download and print out.

RACE	CLASS	RELIGION
GENDER IDENTITY	AGE	EDUCATION
SEXUAL ORIENTATION	(DIS)ABILITY	ETHNICITY
PHYSICAL HEALTH	CITIZENSHIP	GEOGRAPHIC LOCATION
HOUSING	FAMILY HISTORY	SENSE OF BELONGING
LANGUAGE	MENTAL HEALTH	FERTILITY
NATIONAL ORIGIN	NATIONALITY	HERITAGE
OCCUPATION	CULTURE	COMMUNITY
PRIVILEGE	DOMINATION	MARGINALISED
	RACIAL IDENTITY	

My body and me

Natasha D'Aguiar and Kristina Stamatiou

Your client's body has been through trials and tribulations starting from conception through birth to the present day. Our bodies are always changing, whether this is changing weight, elasticity, growing through puberty or menopause or growing fingernails and hair, growing cells.

This activity is for the client to explore their body through art and to begin a conversation about the journey their body has taken. It will give the client a chance to pause and reflect on their relationship with the body they inhabit.

EXPLORING YOUR BODY THROUGH IDENTITY AND CULTURE (60 MINUTES)

Aim: To explore the client's body and their identity, culture and the wider society of which they are a part.

What you will need: Clay or 3D materials, paper and a pen or pencil.

For the client (25 minutes): Let's start with a body scan (see Chapter 4 for the script).

What has your body been called? List all the names your body has been called, whether personally or more generally within society.

Now list everything you say to your own body, either out loud or internally.

Physically feel your body. Starting with your feet, touch, pat and squeeze them. Now work upwards to your ankles, your legs, pelvis, hips, torso, breasts, shoulders, arms, hands, face, head. Move your body in a way that feels okay for you, for example stretch, hug, move around the room or a chair.

What does this feel like? Does your body feel different to before? How has it physically changed? Has your relationship with your body changed over time?

Artmaking (25 minutes): Using clay or 3D materials, make and sculpt a version of your body. This doesn't have to be literal. It can be the whole body or part of it that resonates most with you at this time.

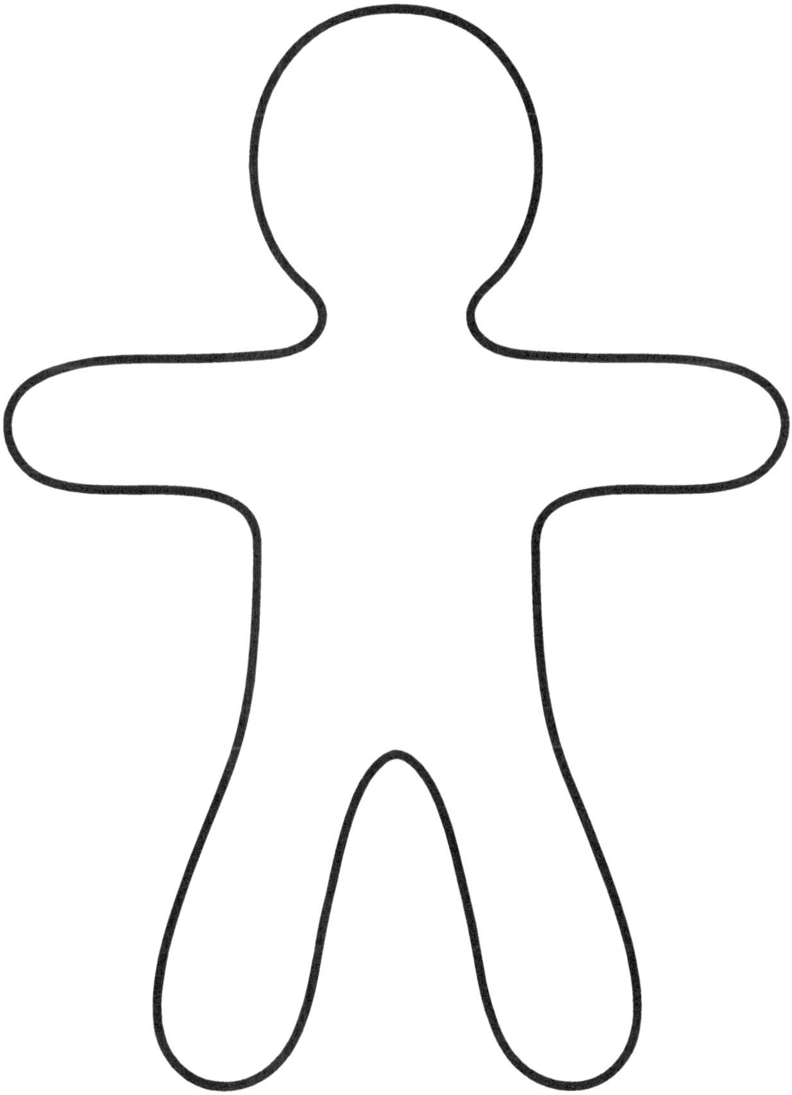

Reflections and questions for the client (10 minutes)

- Looking at your lists from the beginning of the session and looking at your body (or a part of your body), discuss what you would tell your body. Tell your clay or 3D creation what it needs to hear, what it needs, what it is looking for, how it has survived up until now. What are its strengths?
- Thinking about your clay or 3D creation, how has it survived in your culture, in its environment? Does it have a gender?
- How old is it? Is this different to your current age?
- Explore the client's thoughts and feelings around their creation.

Where am I?

Kristina Stamatiou and Natasha D'Aguiar

Explain to the client that they are part of the world they inhabit, contributing to the environment with their presence, taking from the world in each breath and giving back with each exhale. This activity can be done outside or inside.

FINDING YOURSELF (30 MINUTES)

Aim: For the client to connect to their surroundings and the environment they live in.

What you will need: Outdoor space, found objects and glue, scissors and tape.

Outside

For the client: Go for a 5-minute walk around your local environment. While walking, look and feel what's around you. Feel the ground beneath you, take in how it feels beneath your body. Have a go at touching it, smelling it. Look above you. What can you see? Can you feel the elements on the skin? Can you feel warmth, cold, wind or rain? Are there people around you? Close your eyes (if this feels safe for you). What can you hear? Sounds from humans or the environment? Are there any smells in the air?

What season is it? How has this impacted the environment you are in? Take a moment to reflect on this by looking at what's around you. Is it Autumn/Winter? Is there death of trees surrounding you? Are there signs of Spring? Can you see growth?

Select at least five objects. They may stand out to you, or they may not. Maybe they want to be chosen. With your five found objects laid out in front of you, create an image or sculpture (20 minutes).

Reflections and questions for the client (5 minutes)

- What comes up for you when you look at your creation?
- How do you connect with your current environment? Does this differ from anywhere you have lived before?
- Does your environment reflect your class, and if so, how?
- What connection do you have to your surroundings? Does this form part of your identity and who you are?

Inside

If movement in an outdoor space is not available to you, find objects in the room or space you inhabit. Spend 5 minutes looking around the room, feeling what's around you. Feel the different textures, weights, surfaces. Listen to your senses...what do you hear, see and taste?

Select at least five objects from your surroundings. Lay them in front of you. Consider if there is a relationship between each object (20 minutes).

Reflections and questions for the client (5 minutes)

- What comes up for you when you look at your creation?
- How do you connect with your current environment? Does this differ from anywhere you have lived before?
- Does your environment reflect your class, and if so, how?
- What connection do you have to your surroundings? Does this form part of your identity and who you are?

Inhabiting another body

Kristina Stamatiou and Natasha D'Aguiar

This activity enables the client to connect and explore their body in a creative way, to reflect on how their gender, sexuality, appearance and race is viewed in wider society and in their family relationships.

INHABITING ANOTHER BODY (30 MINUTES)

Aim: For the client to explore their body by inhabiting another while bringing them closer to the limits of their own skin.

What you will need: Internet access or magazines or newspapers, large sheets of paper, pens, poster paints and scissors and tape.

For the client (5 minutes): Take a few minutes to find a body by searching online, using social media or looking through magazines or newspapers. Select a body you are drawn to in any way. This doesn't have to be your ideal body – it can be abstract or figurative. Try not to judge your choice here.

Once you have chosen a body, using the art materials, make it. Be experimental here – it doesn't have to look exactly like the body you have chosen and, again, it can be abstract (10 minutes).

Now you have finished your 'other' body, it's time to embody it.

Walk around the room or move in your space carrying your creation with you. Now move in the way you think the body moves. Moving your fingers, arms, legs, if this is accessible for you – moving fast, then slow. Move your eyes in a way the body's eyes may move. Move your breath in a way the body may breathe – is their breath faster or slower than your own? Experiment with making sounds the body may make (5 minutes).

Reflections and questions for the client (10 minutes)

- How does it feel to inhabit another body? What are the similarities and differences to your own body? Is it human, is it hairy or smooth?
- What sort of life does this body have?
- Think about the other body's life – whether they work and what experiences they've had. What race or heritage is it? Does it have a gender?
- What changes when you inhabit another body? What feels different? How would others respond to a body such as this?

Voice

Kristina Stamatiou and Natasha D'Aguiar

This activity can touch on class, heritage, ethnicity and gender.

USING YOUR VOICE (30 MINUTES)

Aim: To explore identity through voice, music and sound.

What you will need: Recording device, e.g., phone, laptop, sheet of paper and a pen.

For the client (10 minutes): Explore your voice and how you sound. Make a noise in any way that feels comfortable to you. Exploring the loudness of your voice, make loud noises, and now make quiet sounds. How loud can your voice go? How quiet can you be? This could be in terms of your accent or vocal tone or pitch. Record your voice on a device [the therapist may also do this]. After playing both recordings back out loud, reflect with the therapist on what this experience is like. What are the similarities and differences between your voices? Do they clash or sound harmonious together? Explore this together.

Using a piece of paper, write a list of people in your network who sound similar to you (10 minutes).

Consider your voice, accent, language, etc., and compare this to your family members, your peers and people at your work (or school). Notice where your vocal peers are and how this feels while also noticing where the differences lie.

Reflections and questions for the client (10 minutes)

- How did it feel to explore your voice?
- What discoveries did you make about where your voice intersects identity in terms of class, heritage and gender?
- How has your voice changed over time?

- Perhaps you speak different languages – how does your voice change when you speak in different languages?
- How loud or quiet are you? Do you sneeze or cough in a particular volume? Does this connect to your speaking voice?
- Do you breathe loudly, quietly, etc.?

A collaboration of two worlds: Exploring your world using art

Kristina Stamatiou and Natasha D'Aguiar

Here we use the word 'world' as a metaphor to describe the client's life. Our worlds all look different, depending on where we live, the people we live with and how we enjoy spending our time. There will be similarities and differences within all our relationships and the worlds of which we are a part. We may feel as though we need to make our world smaller in order to fit in with other people's worlds. Does the world you would like to live in exist? Does the world in which you currently live take into account your needs?

Some of us take part in daily rituals, some of us listen to music, enjoy a shower or a bath, some like to cook, clean, read, dance, etc....we may like quiet or we may like noise...all these things are part of our world. There may be times when our needs or likes are not taken into account in the physical world.

We encourage co-production with the client for this activity.

UNDERSTANDING OUR WORLD (50 MINUTES)

Aim: To help the client reflect and understand their world.

What you will need: Paper, scissors, coloured pens or pencils and glue.

Part 1 (approx. 5 minutes)

With the client, cut out two round circles from a piece of paper (you can also use an online medium for this). These two round circles will act as your own worlds – one world should be given to the client and one world should remain with you.

Part 2 (15 minutes)

Together with the client, make a list on separate pieces of paper of what is important to have in your world. These can be people, places, spaces, objects, rituals, activities, certain shops...

Make a list of which you wished you had less of in your world, what you do not want to be part of your world.

Finally, make a list of your needs within your world – for example, would you want your world to be quieter, more playful...?

Part 3 (25 minutes)

Write or draw your lists on to your worlds – be as playful and as creative as you like, using words, images, symbols and colours, etc.

Reflections and questions for both therapist and client (5 minutes)

Stop the artmaking and have a look at what you have both created. Notice any similarities and any differences between your worlds – have you used the same colours, similar shapes or words...? Be curious around these similarities and differences...

- What was it like creating your world in a visual way?
- What was it like thinking about what you wanted to put on your world?
- What was it like thinking about what you did not want as part of your world?
- Explain how it would be like if you lived on this world.
- What have you noticed about each other's world?
- What was it like sharing your worlds with each other?

Cultural map

Kristina Stamatiou and Natasha D'Aguiar

Maps are guides that show us where we are going and where we have been. They show main roads, acres of land and also the small bendy roads that may feel insignificant. This activity is a way to visually represent various aspects of the self, including, and not limited to, race, culture, environment, class, ability, education, employment, relationships, pregnancy, religion, spirituality, sexuality, age and gender.

Using the map as a metaphor, the client will be invited to map out their identity on the piece of paper.

CREATING A CULTURAL MAP (50 MINUTES)

Aim: To take the client on a journey of exploration and reflection, bringing awareness to certain parts of their identity, highlighting those that take a back seat.

What you will need: One sheet of A4 paper and one sheet of A3 paper and dry art materials, such as colouring pencils, felt tip pens or oil pastels or soft pastels.

Part 1 (5–10 minutes)

For the client: On the A4 sheet of paper write a list of parts of your identity that first come to mind. Take a few minutes to complete this. You do not need to write everything – just the first things that come to mind.

Part 2 (30 minutes)

For the client: On the A3 sheet of paper, begin to draw a symbol, mark or character for each part of your identity you listed in Part 1. Plot these across the paper in any way that feels right for you.

Consider how each symbol or mark interacts with each other – for example are they separate, or are they joined up?

Reflections and questions for the client (10 minutes)

- How did it feel to list parts of your identity?
- What is missing, or is there anything that appears very small on the paper?
- What takes up the most space?
- How does each symbol or mark interact with each other?
- What do you notice most?
- What surprises you most about your cultural map?
- Is there anything you would like to add or take away? If so, what would this be?
- What do you notice in your body when looking at your cultural map now? How does it look as a whole?

Connecting to your soul

Kristina Stamatiou and Natasha D'Aguiar

Artmaking is a way to express yourself on a deeper level than the often superficial, day-to-day self-expression we may present to the world in our everyday life, which may get lost. Maybe your client struggles to know who they truly are as they may battle with who they want to be or who they are expected to be. This process aims to reconnect the client with their inner self, their soul, in a holistic way.

CONNECTING TO YOUR INNER SOUL (45 MINUTES)

Aim: For the client to connect to the inner parts of their soul, connecting to their identity, exploring their culture and heritage, and who they truly are on a deeper level.

What you will need: Sheets of A2 paper, paints, a paint brush or palette knife and oil pastels or soft pastels.

For the client (30 minutes): Using a large sheet of paper and a paint colour of your choice, make a mark on the page. This can be any mark, but try to make it stretch from one side of the paper to the other side, filling the space. Now cover the paper using the paints in any way that feels right for you, bearing in mind your soul, who you are and how connected you feel to the world you live in. You may want to think about your intersections and how this makes up part of who you are. Don't think too consciously about what you are painting here – it's important to paint as freely as possible.

There is an option here to list your 'social graces' (5 minutes).

Reflections and questions for the client (10 minutes)

- What was that experience like for you?

- Which of the 'social graces' came up for you? (See Chapter 1 to remind yourself of the 'social graces'.)
- What came to mind as you were painting?
- Does your painting look surprising to you? If so, why?
- How does it feel when you look at your painting?
- What makes you unique?

CHAPTER 4

Exploring Culture and Identity through Words and Movement

Poetic enquiry – Exploring identity and culture

Roula-Maria Dib, scholar and poet

I am a London-based Lebanese-American. I am Levantine (of Antiochian Greek ancestry), and have lived in the USA, Saudi Arabia, Lebanon, United Arab Emirates and the UK. I am a mother, writer, poet and scholar whose interests lie at the interstices of literature, analytical psychology and creativity in general.

According to the French philosopher Gaston Bachelard (1958):

> We comfort ourselves by reliving memories of protection. Something closed must retain our memories, while leaving them their original value as images. Memories of the outside world will never have the same tonality as those of home and, by recalling these memories, we add to our store of dreams; we are never real historians, but always near poets, and our emotion is perhaps nothing but an expression of a poetry that was lost.

The concept of 'home' is often tied to the complexities of the self and the notions of comfort and belonging; it is in constant questioning and exploration, especially among 'global citizens' and those living in the diaspora. As Bachelard suggests, getting in touch with these memories of home can be a poetic act. However, in the following activity, we will explore identity by invoking memories beyond the realm of images.

And we will start the quest from the kitchen. Traditional food, whether cooked or consumed, is a performance of our cultural memory through all our five senses. It can empower our sense of belonging while bringing to the surface and crystallising many aspects of our identity. So much of who we are lies somewhere within the parenthetical womb of taste and memory. By the end of the poem, your client will be surprised by how much of their personal narrative revolves around food, and how much of their personal and cultural maquette is formed in their pantry.

This activity creates a different kind of found poetry. While found poems usually require extracting words or phrases from a text, this activity lets the client extract ingredients from their pantry. Please ask them to come prepared for this activity, possibly exploring the above prior to the session.

POETIC INGREDIENTS (60 MINUTES)

Aim: To explore the concept of home through sensory memory, using food as a gateway to identity, belonging and cultural experience. By reflecting on ingredients and culinary traditions, participants will uncover personal narratives embedded in taste, smell and memory. The exercise encourages creative expression through poetry, allowing individuals to connect with their past and present. Ultimately, it seeks to reveal how deeply food shapes one's sense of self and cultural heritage in unexpected and meaningful ways.

What you will need: Pen and paper.

Part 1 (20 minutes)

For the client: Before the session, go to your pantry, preferably focusing on ingredients that belong to your native cuisine. If you either don't cook or don't have traditional foodstuff in your kitchen, you may want to explore something different, like a menu or a cookbook. [If your client has not been able to do this before the session, please ask them to close their eyes and imagine their pantry.]

Look at the items, and in the manner of a 'found poem', write a list of the first 10 items you spot or spotted.

Every item is a symbol, but it is up to you to assign its symbolic meaning:

- What does the item mean to you?
- Is there a special memory associated with it (an event, a friend, a family member...)?
- Does it have a certain cultural significance (your country, religion, hometown, tradition, myth...)?
- Does it have a representational quality (something in the colour, shape, taste, etc.)? Think of each item's symbolic significance.

For example: Rose water = grandmother, native rose bushes in your hometown, Aphrodite's tears, red, sweetness, distillation.

Put these items in your list into pairs. This can be done randomly, but if you find particular ingredients that blend well together in cooking (like oil and vinegar, for example), couple them up. The opposite worlds of oil and vinegar reflect the two sides of truth: mystery and the clarity.

Look more closely at the 'bonding force' in each pair – think of an analogical relationship between the two items. They can be opposites of each other, complementary, similar, joined by a common factor, etc.

Write one sentence (or more) talking about the relationship between the two items in each pair and the images that arise as you write about it. The sentences don't have to be complete – they can just be phrases. Here's an example (for rose water and a bottle of red wine):

> A Mediterranean summer is sweet like rose cordial and long like the bottle of Syrah wine; Aphrodite's tears are in one bottle and her blood in the other.

Part 2 (20 minutes)

For the client: You will have worked up quite a few sentences by the end of the fifth pair. And by now, many images and memories would have arisen. Are there any people, characters or even natural elements that you may like to create a dialogue with? Choose one.

Whether you have chosen to converse with Poseidon, a grandparent, a rose bush or even a mountain, take 10 minutes (at least – allow more time if needed) to do some active imagination. During these 10 minutes, you may want to write down your dialogue as it happens spontaneously.

Here are some starter questions:

- Why are you here?
- What do you bring me?
- How are we alike?

Then ask this character for a favour. Be as daring as you can!

Part 3 (20 minutes)

For the client: Go back to the material you wrote in Part 1. Arrange the sentences into stanzas. You should have five, one for each pair of ingredients. Be as economic as possible with the words, so focus on letting the verses show rather than tell, so anything cliché or redundant may need to be eliminated. Leave in the things you discovered or that you came up with during the writing process.

Go to the material you wrote in Part 2. Look at the questions and the answers from the dialogue (but hold on to the favour you asked for in your final question). Spread them out at the end of each stanza. You may, for example, choose to write one or two verses at the end and also include something from the dialogue in other locations of the stanzas.

By the time the first draft of the poem is completed, you will be surprised by how much 'identity material' you have learned and connected with!

Identity exploration using poetry

Kristina Stamatiou

Poetry can be an expressive and powerful means to delve into a person's identity using creativity. Poetry can be used to help explore our inner emotions, truths and complexities, which are associated with our identity.

This activity will ask the client to think about their own identity, whether this be their heritage, gender, religion or beliefs, sexuality, appearance, class, disability, etc....

IDENTITY PLAY (50 MINUTES)

Aim: To help the client explore their own identity using poetry.

What you will need: Pen and paper or an online writing document.

Part 1 (15 minutes)

For the client: Using a pen and paper or an online writing document, make a list of four truths about you and your identity. This could be around your appearance, sexuality, relationship status, gender, class, etc.... Once you have a list of these four truths, next to each truth write a colour that you feel is connected to the truth. Once you have your four truths and four colours, write next to the colours an animal that you feel connects to the truth and colour. Finally write a number that you feel drawn to next to the truth. You should have something that reads as follows:

> Woman, Green, Crow, 7

Once you have finished, create four false truths about you. This can be linked to anything that was once told to you about your identity. Was there anything someone may have said about you that is not true? Has the media ever said anything about your identity that you can remember which is not true? Now create your four false truths using the same process as above – connect a colour, an animal and a number to your false truths. For example:

> Thunder, Yellow, Sheep, 5

Part 2 (30 minutes)

For the client: Now that you have your lists of truths and false truths with supporting colours, animals and numbers, you are going to begin to write a poem. To start the poem please pick one truth and its associated colour, animal and number along with one false truth with its associated colour, animal and number. Create a sentence that you feel connects them together. When exploring identity in this way, you can be as creative as possible with your language and sentence. For example:

> The woman across the road draws green thunder from her apple.

> As seven crows pick yellow feathers from a sheep's back...

Now you have the opening lines of your poem, continue to use up the truths and false truths in the same way as you did to complete your poem.

Reflections and questions for the client (5 minutes)

Ask the client if they would like to share their poem with you. They can either read it aloud themselves or you can read it for them. Please negotiate with the client what feels best for them. They may also not want to share their poem, and that is okay. Here are some questions you can ask your client about this creative writing activity:

- How did your body feel while you were writing your four truths?
- How did your body feel while you were writing your four false truths?
- What part of the writing process did you find most difficult?

- How does it feel to write a poem around these truths and false truths?
- How did it feel to read your poem aloud?
- How did it feel for me, your therapist, to read/listen to the poem?

Exploring identity through creative writing

Kristina Stamatiou and Natasha D'Aguiar

Letter writing can be therapeutic. With the client, consider what it feels like to send and receive post. It can help to externalise yourself and think about your future self and speak to them. In this activity the client writes a letter to their future self – exploring what they would tell their future self, where they would like to be in the future and how they would want life to look. Who do they want to be and what would need to change around them and within them to make this shift? Do parts of their identity need to change, or does society need to change to accept them? With the client, reflect on which aspects of themselves feel unacceptable, which parts they quieten that they may like to be louder. Remind them of the 'social graces' model (see Chapter 1).

A CONVERSATION WITH FUTURE ME (30 MINUTES)

Aim: To consider your future self by reflecting on the social graces. Participants will explore how identity, relationships and life experiences may evolve across family, social, professional and spiritual domains. Through letter writing, the exercise encourages empathy, self-awareness and intentional thinking about hopes, challenges and growth, supporting a deeper understanding of personal values and possible futures.

What you will need: Pen and paper or an online writing document.

For the client (5 minutes): List the 'social graces' to begin the conversation with yourself, in keeping with all aspects of intersectionality.

Consider what your future self might hope for and dream about. They may have experienced loss, love, happiness, hopefulness, despair. How do you imagine their family life, social life, work life and spiritual life? Use this template to complete your own letter (15 minutes):

Dear [add name]

I am [add age] years old and I imagine you are [add age] years old.

Currently I'm doing/feeling [family, social life, work, mental and physical health, wellbeing, e.g., I am married with one child; I have a valued friendship group that I don't see as often as I'd like but speak to regularly; My mental health can improve as my anxiety sometimes gets the better of me; My physical health is getting better, my pain is under control] [add]

I'm grateful for [add]

You may have experienced [add]

I hope you are [add]

I predict you [family, social life, work, mental and physical health, wellbeing, e.g., I predict you will have more children and are still happily married, that you have friendships and have continued making new ones; Your mental health has improved; although you may still have anxious feelings, this doesn't stop you from doing what you want in life; You continue to manage your physical pain and find time to exercise when you can; Your general wellbeing is stable as you have a strong support circle] [add]

[Sign off]

Reflections and questions for the client (10 minutes)

- What did this bring up for you?
- How do you feel about your future self compared to your current life?
- Are there many differences? If so, what are these?

Colour-out poem

Kristina Stamatiou and Natasha D'Aguiar

Creating colour-out poems can provide a playful way to be creative with words. It can set us free from self-criticism as we only have limited words that the text gives us, thus allowing the writers to free themselves from some judgement.

WRITING A COLOUR-OUT POEM (30 MINUTES)

Aim: To use ready-made prose to create a poem in an unconscious free-flowing way to explore various aspects of intersectionality. This is dependent on the client, the text they choose and what comes up in their poem.

What you will need: Newspaper, magazine or electronic device and a dark colour (black) felt tip pen.

For the client (5 minutes): Select an article from a newspaper or magazine that means something to you and reflects who you are in some way (keep in mind what source the client may bring and what this may reflect about their cultural context).

Poem (15 minutes): Now you have selected an article, create a poem by selecting one word per line, selecting a word that stands out to you, and then delete the other words by colouring them in with a black pen or equivalent on your electronic device. Your chosen words do not need to make grammatical sense. Try to be as free-flowing as possible and select the word that you're attracted to the most.

Once you have come to the end of the article, read your poem out loud.

Reflections and questions for the client (10 minutes)

- Does your chosen newspaper or magazine reflect your class, gender, race or where you were educated?
- Does it reflect your age or cultural background or any other parts of your identity?
- What came up for you in your poem?
- What was it like to read your poem out loud with a witness?

Myth and storytelling

Kristina Stamatiou

Myths and storytelling have played an important role in my childhood. The majority of my childhood memories rest on my grandad's constant storytelling. As my mother prepared the dinner table, my grandad would begin; whether he would be recalling a memory based on a true event, a historical event or a myth that had been passed on through generations, it took centre stage of our dinner conversations. The myth or story would always serve a purpose with a deeper symbolic or metaphorical meaning.

This activity can also be explored during online therapy, using an online medium such as a writing document. I have chosen to share a traditional Cypriot myth with you (see below).

SHARING A MYTH OR STORY (60 MINUTES)

Aim: To explore personal and cultural identity through storytelling by engaging with myths and their symbolic meanings. By reflecting on familial or adapted myths, participants are encouraged to uncover deeper narratives about heritage, beliefs and values. The exercise fosters curiosity, interpretation and creative expression, supporting a richer understanding of how stories shape identity, connection and a sense of belonging across generations and cultures.

What you will need: Pens or felt tip pens and paper.

Part 1 (5–10 minutes)

Please read the myth aloud to your client and use it as a base to wonder with your client about any familial myths that they may have been told. Ask them to share the myth, and wonder with them about any symbolic or metaphorical meaning their myth is sharing. Alternatively, if they cannot think of any myths themselves, ask them to adapt this Cypriot myth in a way that may feel more relevant to their own heritage.

A Cypriot myth of the olive tree

The olive tree is considered a sacred tree in Cyprus. It not only provides an income for the island due to its glorious olive oil, but it also holds a spiritual value. The olive tree's sacredness has been based on an old folk tale. It has been said that the olive tree hid Jesus to protect him, and in turn, the olive tree was blessed with longevity. The olive tree asks Jesus, 'What happens if someone cuts me down?' Jesus replies and tells the tree that their olive leaves and branches will produce smoke, which will burn, and in turn keep the tree safe from evil and envy. This folk tale is still celebrated by many Cypriots to this day. They often burn olive leaves in incense burners to bless their homes, families and friends. The ritual is also used in churches, for weddings, christenings and funerals. It is not only used for Christian Cypriots but also for Muslim Cypriots on the island who also view the olive burning ritual as a form of protection and blessing.

Part 2 (25 minutes)

Ask your client to think of their own experiences with myths. Wonder with them if they have ever heard their families share any stories or myths with them. Ask them to write down this myth or story they remember on their sheet of paper or online document. They could also include drawing and images when documenting their myth or story.

Reflections and questions for the client (25 minutes)

- Do you remember how old you were when you first heard this myth?
- What family member, friend or person shared this myth with you?
- What is the symbolic or metaphorical meaning behind the myth?
- How does it feel to write the myth down?
- Do you feel connected to this myth, and if so, why?

- If you could change or adapt the myth so that you could feel more connected to it, what section would you adapt?
- Reflect with your client about this process. Ask them how this activity felt for them. If they would like to, they can draw their reflections or write down a few words on a piece of paper.

Myth within dramatherapy

Grace Linstead, Sesame dramatherapist

What makes up my identity? This question went around in my head when I was asked to contribute to this wonderful book. I am a woman, I am a daughter, I am a wife, I am a friend, I am a sister, I am a dramatherapist (and, as I explore later on within this piece of writing, I am a Sesame dramatherapist)... This served as a reminder for me that we all have many different 'roles' we play that make up our identity and our character, and that we are all the main character of our own life story. Then, the word 'story' stuck with me.

Storytelling, story making and work with myth and fairy tale are creative ways of helping our clients to explore their identity within a group or one-to-one dramatherapy session. When facilitating a myth session with their client(s), the dramatherapist tells a story within the session that relates to the client(s) in some way, a story whose message might be healing for the client(s). The therapist and client(s) can then choose to explore this story in some way, whether this be physically through enactment, or through other creative means (drawing, writing, movement, etc.).

Finding your own personal myth was something that was integral to the Dramatherapy Master's training I completed in 2019. The 'Myth assessment', which every student must complete during the UK HCPC-registered Dramatherapy Master's, requires the student to facilitate a myth session with the rest of the cohort acting as clients. The trainee dramatherapist who is being assessed is encouraged to pick a story they feel connected with, and which links to their identity.

Joseph Campbell writes how powerful and beneficial myths can be for an individual: 'when the story is in your mind, then you see its relevance to something happening in your own life. It gives you perspective on what is happening to you' (Campbell 1991, p.2).

The Dramatherapy Master's I completed followed the Sesame approach, which follows the teachings of Marian 'Billy' Lindkvist, who developed the branch of dramatherapy called 'Sesame'. Sesame dramatherapy recognises the importance of myth and fairy tale within the therapeutic space, and also Laban Movement Analysis (LMA) (a method and language for describing, visualising, interpreting and documenting human movement) and movement with touch and sound, as written about in the aptly-named chapter 'Speech Doesn't Count – Much' in her book. A Sesame dramatherapist ensures that 'the emphasis is on the development of the person as a whole through the creative experience' (Lindkvist 1998, p.259). Sesame, its structure and its magic, forms another branch of my identity as a Sesame-trained dramatherapist, and underpins any session I facilitate with my clients.

FACILITATING A MYTH SESSION (USING THE SESAME DRAMATHERAPY STRUCTURE) (60 MINUTES)

Check-in (5 minutes): Invite the client to express how they are feeling today in a creative way (e.g., by using a sound and movement, a drawing, or by picking an object).

Warm-up (5 minutes): Invite the client to engage in a game to bring 'play' into the space.

Bridge in (10 minutes): Invite the client to engage in an activity which links to the themes of the story you are about to tell them (e.g., if you are telling the story of Cinderella, you could invite the client to imaginatively explore the castle with you, or imaginatively 'try on' different pairs of shoes and walk around and explore what kind of characters come out of wearing these shoes).

Main event (20 minutes): Tell the client the story and invite any reflections or enactments or explorations of the story. They could enact the whole story or just one section or character they relate to the most. You could also invite the client to draw, paint or creatively write this part of the story.

Bridge out (10 minutes): Invite the client to amplify these reflections. Is there one theme or character within the story that resonates most with them that they want to focus on? They could create a character profile for this character or verbally explain what this theme means to them. An important part of the 'Bridge out' is also to 'travel out' of the story space and come back to the present and to reality (e.g., for the story of Cinderella, travelling out of the castle and away from the castle grounds, and coming back to the room where the session is taking place).

Grounding (5 minutes): Invite the client to engage in activities which ground them.

Reflections and questions for the client (5 minutes)

- Which character in the story do you relate to the most, and why?
- What friends or family members do you see in any of the characters within the story?
- Which is your favourite part of the story?
- What reflections do you have on the story?
- How do you feel about the story/the character/the themes?
- What message would you like to tell a certain character in the story?
- If the story had another name or title, what would it be?
- What could an alternative ending be to the story?

I hope this is helpful in giving you the confidence to embrace the wonders of myth, fairy tale and Sesame dramatherapy when working with your clients, whether that be in group or one-to-one therapy sessions: 'Myths and stories offer an experience which every participant is free to feel and interpret in their own way, according to how it feels in the doing. That way the story never loses its capacity to surprise' (Gersie, quoted in Pearson, Smail and Watts 2013, pp.20–21).

Exploring identity through dance and movement

Emma Fisher, dance movement psychotherapist

> *Why do I dance? Dance is my medicine. It's the scream which eases for a while the terrible frustration common to all human beings who because of race, creed, or color, are 'invisible'. Dance is the fist with which I fight the sickening ignorance of prejudice.*
>
> PEARL PRIMUS, AMERICAN DANCER, CHOREOGRAPHER AND ANTHROPOLOGIST (TAKEN FROM SCHWARTZ AND SCHWARTZ 2011)

Dancing and moving is for everybody. It is especially for those bodies whom, because of the intersections of their identities, society has subjugated and oppressed. If you have a body and you have breath, you are moving, and if you move, there is capacity for expression and communication through movement.

Our stories are woven into the fabric of our bodies – our muscles and our bones – and on a very cellular level. And not just our individual stories. The body is inhabited by generations of family relationships (Govoni and Weatherhogg 2007). On a cellular level, our bodies and our nervous systems hold the stories of our families passed down through generations. Stories of our culture, the societies we live in and they lived in, and the world events experienced sitting alongside our own lived experiences – all these narratives weaving an intricate textile that can at times be difficult to untangle.

Dancing is the act of taking these internal stories of the body and externalising them, making them visible for a fleeting moment to those around us. The being moved from within and sharing it beyond the boundaries of our own self.

Not only can movement help us share and make sense of our experiences; it can also help us to re-choreograph our narratives of self, our relationship to our body, and change the shape of the genetic material we pass on to our next generations.

I discovered dancing at the age of three, in Australia. My passion and pursuit of dancing moved me from Australia to Germany at the age of 15, eventually settling me in London. As a white, cisgender, athletically built, able-bodied woman, I have the privilege of inhabiting the type of body that society views as acceptable, including as acceptable for it to be seen and expressed in movement.

Many of the bodies we meet in therapy will not have had this experience.

Despite the inherent privilege I hold, myself, my appearance and my body also experience sexualisation by a society with a dominant male gaze. I am subjugated by sexism and misogyny and carry the lived experiences of abuse that remind me of this.

There are many other forms of oppression of the body that may interact with our and our clients' identities: racism, ableism, classism, ageism, fatphobia, homophobia and heteronormativity. These inform the discourses about bodies and movement and may lead us to modulate how we occupy and move our bodies. Dance involves the body, emotion and mind. All three of these are culturally mediated, not only biologically based. Our perceptions and use of body, emotion and mind are influenced by culture (Hanna 1988). We can reclaim a sense of bodily autonomy by reconnecting to our bodies and integrating them as part of our identity.

Movement is communication. When we are born forth into the world it is the first way we communicate our desires, our needs, our fears. Movement and sensory experiences and how they are understood and fed back to us in the early phases of our lives provide the foundation for empathy, communication, emotional regulation and the emotional understanding that we carry with us for the rest of our lives. This is our first dance, the dance of relating.

This knowledge is stored as wordless stories, including stories about what is safe and what might be dangerous in the world around us. We all carry this implicit early experience within our bodies, and creative movement is one of the ways we can come to understand more about the experiences we hold, and how we can share them with others.

Movement allows us to express that which is beyond words, or comes from a time before we had the words to make sense of our experiences. This movement activity offers an invitation for clients and therapists to tune into the stories held within the physical fabric of the body, and to begin to explore the intersectional threads that are woven into it.

DISCOVERING NEW STORIES (60 MINUTES)

Aim: Connecting to the wordless stories of the body and narratives of self in the context of intersectionality.

What you will need: A chair.

You may like to provide music to offer containment, or ask the client to contribute music that is meaningful to them.

Lead the client through the body scan script (see below), to offer grounding and prepare them to use movement in an exploratory way.

Invite them to bring to mind an aspect of their identity (2–3 minutes).

Offer an invitation to allow that part of themselves to mould their body into a position that feels right. They may like to take some time exploring different bodily shapes, until one lands in the body. They may also like to explore different spatial configurations within the room (5 minutes).

Ask them to notice what this shape feels like, and any metaphors or images that come to mind.

Now invite them to bring to mind another aspect of their intersectional identity (2–3 minutes).

Repeat the invitation to allow that part of themselves to shape their body. You can offer this invitation as many times as feels meaningful to the client (5 minutes).

Then, invite them to move between these different bodily shapes and forms, creating a dance that weaves together the different aspects of their identity (10 minutes).

Reflections and questions for the client (15 minutes)

- What thoughts, images or metaphors arise as you allow each aspect of your identity to shape your body?
- Is there a difference in how the positions feel in your body?

- Do you have a sense of what internal or external assumptions or judgements might be leading to these different feelings? If so, please explain.
- What is it like to have me, your therapist, witness these different parts of you, your identity?
- What parts of your body hold power or privilege?
- What parts of your body are often overlooked, ignored or subjugated? By yourself and/or others?
- What do you notice about what is needed to move between these different parts of yourself? Are some of them easier to move between than others?
- Which parts of yourself have you found yourself ignoring in this creative process?
- As a therapist, notice how you witness these movements, how you experience them in your own body, and how your body may want to react or respond in the position of witness.

Body scan script (20 minutes)

Find a comfortable position in a chair. If you can, try and have your feet flat on the ground.

Begin by taking in the space around you. You might notice the sounds in the room, the temperature of the air.

Take a moment to notice your breath, your heartbeat – the rhythms of the body which connect us all.

Lean back against the back of your chair. Feel the support of the chair behind you.

Now bring the attention to your feet and the ground beneath them. The ground that is always there, to support us. Feeling the support of the earth beneath you, you may wish to welcome some movement into your feet.

Wiggle your toes.

Rock gently from the back of your foot to the front, exploring connection to the floor with your toes, then your heels.

Bring your attention up from your feet, through the calves and shins...through the back of your legs.

Bring your attention all the way up the back. Noticing the

support of the chair behind you, begin to gently move your back. Maybe gently swaying from side to side. Feeling and exploring the support in different parts of your back. Noticing where your back has contact with the chair and the support it offers, and where it doesn't.

Now, we bring our attention to your shoulders. Gently squeezing them up toward the ears, and then dropping them back down. Repeat this a few times. You may want to reach out your arms into a big, wide, releasing yawn.

Bringing the hands together in front of you. Give your hands a gentle squeeze. Noticing the support of your own body. Gently squeezing and massaging your hands. Sit back against the back of the chair.

Squeeze your hands, wriggle your fingers, and allow your hands to take a shape that represents where you are at today, what you are arriving with.

CHAPTER 5

Exploring Culture and Identity through Geography, Music and Food

Exploring identity and culture through flags

Kristina Stamatiou and Natasha D'Aguiar

Flags can hold many meanings and interpretations among individuals, communities and nations. Flags can be viewed as symbolic; they may show symbols, colours and shapes that can serve as shared representatives for communities and nations. They can symbolise a collective sense of identity and beliefs. Some flags may also share and hold political ideologies, religious beliefs or even historical events. They can be used in protest and in celebrations, bringing people together expressing solidarity and even asserting their views.

Wonder with the client about their heritage, race, sexuality, gender, disability, religion, etc.... Ask them to think about any flags they are drawn to or any flags that may cause discomfort within their bodies.

WHAT FLAGS MEAN TO YOU (55 MINUTES)

Aim: For the client to think about any flags that they feel represents them and their identity, culture or beliefs.

What you will need: Paper, pens, pencils, paints or felt tip pens and scissors.

Part 1 (10 minutes)

Please ask your client to close their eyes. Ask them to think about any flags they have seen, flags that may represent their heritage or their family's heritage. Now, ask them to think about any flags that are personal to them and their own identity. While keeping their eyes shut, ask your client to visualise these flags, to think about their colours, if there are any symbols on these flags. Finally, ask your client to open their eyes. Get them to write down any colours, shapes or symbols they saw, on a piece of paper.

Part 2 (30 minutes)

Invite your client to create their own flag. Ask them to think about what came up for them in Part 1. Wonder with them whether they could create a unique flag that incorporates their identity and intersections. They can be as creative as they wish with colours, symbols and shapes.

Reflections and questions for the client (10 minutes)

- How did it feel to close your eyes and think of flags you may have previously seen?
- What flags made you feel uncomfortable?
- What flags are you proud of, and why?
- What do flags mean to you?
- How did it feel to create your own flag unique to you and your identity?

Ending (5 minutes)

Finally, ask your client what they would like to do with their flag.

Geography and identity

Kristina Stamatiou and Natasha D'Aguiar

Geography can shape and influence our identity and culture. It can influence our beliefs, educational systems, religion, relationships and experiences. You may have lived in different countries, or moved to different towns and areas within the same country. Geography can also overlap with immigration, displacement and even invisible borders. Moving or migrating to different countries or areas can have an effect on both able bodies and bodies with health conditions or impairments. People may have moved out of free choice or had no other choice because of war or conflict.

Different geographical areas share their own relationship with nature and can influence the relationship that people have with the natural world. Moreover, geography also plays a role in entertainment, how we choose to socialise, or even the music and language we use.

Here we are going to explore the areas where your client has lived, travelled to, moved to, or even where their family has lived. This activity can be adapted and used online with an online creative programme of your choice.

EXPLORING GEOGRAPHY AND IDENTITY (55 MINUTES)

Aim: To explore identity through memory and place by mapping personal journeys across locations. By creating a visual timeline and collage, participants reflect on travel, migration and meaningful environments. The process encourages creativity and self-expression while deepening awareness of how landscapes, transitions and lived experiences contribute to one's evolving sense of self and belonging.

What you will need: Old magazines, newspapers or postcards, found materials or objects, paper and scissors and glue.

Part 1 (15 minutes)

For the client: Create a visual timeline, thinking about all the countries you may have visited, migrated from, different areas you may have moved to. How may you have travelled to these countries or areas? Was it by aeroplane, boat, car, train or any other mode of transport? Do you remember any landmarks that you associate with the area? What was the weather like? What was the nature like? Complete your visual timeline.

Part 2 (20 minutes)

For the client: Now you are going to create a collage using the found materials or objects you have. Thinking about your visual timeline, be as creative as you like; you may want to add words, an image or both.

Reflections and questions for the client (15 minutes)

- When you first thought about the different countries or areas you have moved to, what did you want to do to your body? Did you want to comfort it? If so, how did you want to comfort it?
- Do you feel connected to any areas you have lived in previously or the area in which you currently live? If so, which areas?
- What are the landscapes you associate with the area? How often did you or do you visit them? Is it still possible to visit them now?
- Did you have a favourite place within your previous geographic areas that you visited? If so, which areas?
- What is your favourite area in the current location that you visit?

Ending (5 minutes)

For the client: Finally, close your eyes. Take four deep breaths in and exhale out, counting in your head to five as you do this. Repeat the process five times.

Exploring geographical culture through music

Kristina Stamatiou and Natasha D'Aguiar

Music, geography and culture share an intricate relationship. Geography can influence the diversity of musical genres, musical instruments and even traditions. Different countries and areas within the same country have distinctive musical styles and even distinctive musical instruments. There are many factors within a geographical area which can influence music, such as local culture and environment.

An example of a musical genre is jazz, which originated in the USA, specifically from African American communities, which then saw it spread around the world.

Music can bring people together and help us celebrate our similarities and differences. It can help express our physical, emotional, social and cognitive needs.

EXPLORING MUSIC THROUGH IDENTITY AND CULTURE (50 MINUTES)

Aim: To explore music in terms of the client's own identity and culture.

What you will need: A phone, electronic device or an instrument the client knows how to play.

For the client (10 minutes): Think of five places where you would listen to music, for example in your car, bedroom, a social event or gathering. Now think of five songs you feel connected to. Think about what draws you to these songs. Why do you listen to these songs?

Now go to your play lists or pick up your instrument. Can you play the first 3 minutes of the songs aloud? (20 minutes.)

Reflections and questions for the client (20 minutes)

- Was it difficult choosing what songs you wanted to play? If so, why?
- What drew you to the five songs you picked?
- Do these songs hold any specific memories for you? If so, what are these memories?
- When was the last time you played these songs?
- What specific song connects you to your identity in terms of race, sexuality, gender, disability, spirituality, religion, class, etc....?
- How did it feel to play these songs and have them listened to by me, your therapist?
- Did your body respond differently to the different songs? If so, how?
- Have any of these songs been passed down through family? If so, which ones?
- Would you pass down these songs or play them to others? If so, why?

Food and culture

Kristina Stamatiou and Natasha D'Aguiar

Food is a vital part of our lives. We need food for nutrition and health, to provide us with energy and help our cognitive function. Food is also tied deeply to cultural identity and heritage. Recipes are passed down from generations, in an attempt to preserve cultural traditions and identity, connecting people back to their cultural roots. Cooking and preparing food can be seen as a ritualistic act, a way of grounding and remaining present in the moment.

Different foods are served at different times of the year for some people, and some people fast or break a fast and celebrate with food. For example, Orthodox Christians fasting during Lent will give up meat, fish, dairy, oil and wine for 40 days, although this can vary. Food also brings people together and offers social cohesion.

Financial difficulties and geographical setting also influence what we may be able to cook. It might be difficult for some families to maintain cultural dishes linked to their heritage due to either the unavailability of these products or the financial expense, causing anxiety and stress in some circumstances.

EXPLORING FOOD AND CULTURE (50 MINUTES)

Aim: To creatively explore the client's own relationship with food, thinking about their identity and culture.

What you will need: Paper and pens, pencils or felt tip pens.

Part 1 (15 minutes)

For the client: Close your eyes and imagine you are sitting at a dinner table, with either family, friends, colleagues or a carer. Your dinner is about to be served. Look around the table – who is at the table with you? Who has prepared the dinner...was it you? Is it a specific time of the year? Are you at a celebration or an event? What smells are circulating the space?

Your plate arrives and so do the plates of the others around you. What food is on your plate?

Part 2 (20 minutes)

Here is a circle-shaped plate that you can download, print out and draw on for Part 2 of this activity. Alternatively you can draw your own plate on a separate piece of paper. If you would like to, you can use the dinner plate to complete your creative activity.

For the client: Using either the dinner plate as a guide or drawing your own on a piece of paper, please draw what foods are on your dinner plate, and then complete another plate for the person who joined you at the dinner table. If there was more than one person who joined you for dinner, please draw what food is on their plate too. Are their plates the same as yours, or different?

Reflections and questions for the client (15 minutes)

- Who joined you for dinner?
- How many people were around the dinner table?
- What could you smell coming from your dinner plate?
- Was there anything that made it on to your plate that you don't enjoy eating? If so, what was this?
- Does your plate look different to those around you? If so, why?
- Who was cooking the dinner?
- Have you ever cooked before? If so, what is your relationship with cooking?
- Who used to cook for you when you were younger?
- Who cooks for you now?
- How do you feel when it is approaching dinnertime?

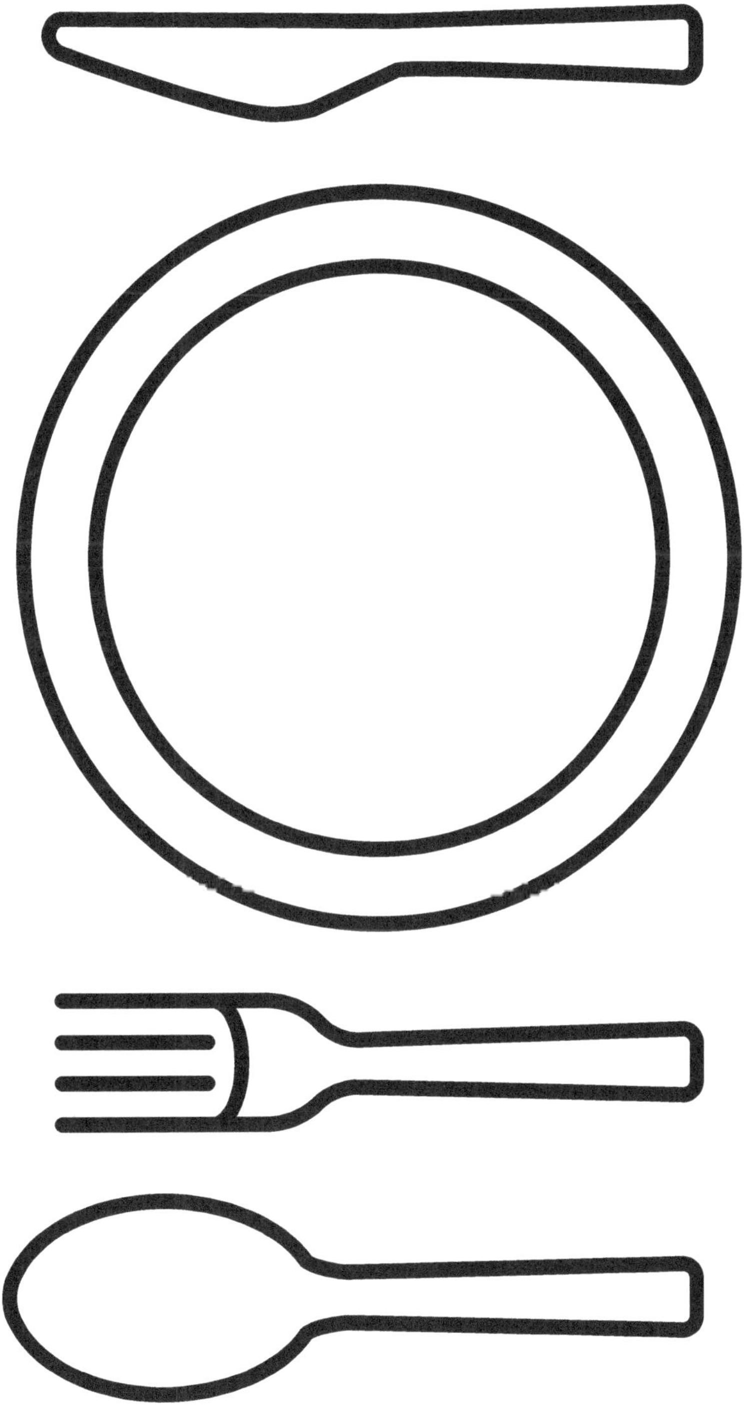

Developmental food

Natasha D'Aguiar and Kristina Stamatiou

This activity explores the client's identity in relation to what they consume and how this may differ throughout their upbringing, exploring the differences and similarities visually. It can be adapted for children, adolescents and adults.

DEVELOPMENTAL FOOD (1 HOUR 20 MINUTES, 2 SESSIONS)

Aim: To explore the client's identity and cultural significance towards food and how this connects with them over their various developmental stages growing up, so they can gain a deeper understanding of themselves.

What you will need: Four sheets of paper, a pen, pencil or electronic device, basic art materials (of the client's choice) and clay.

Session 1 (50 minutes)

For the client: (10 minutes) Let's start with a guided visualisation. I'm going to guide you through from birth to the present day, and how you imagine your future self in connection to the food and drink you consume.

Find a comfortable seat and allow your body to relax. Softly close your eyes, if this feels safe.

Breathe in through your nose for 4 seconds and out through your mouth for 4 seconds. Repeat this breath cycle three times.

With your eyes still closed, take me back to when you were a newborn baby. You're in your home, in your cot, bassinet or wherever you would lay. Perhaps you're in a caregiver's bedroom, living room or in a caregiver's arms. [Pause.]

Notice how you feel in your body. Do you have any physical reactions? Do you notice any changes in your nervous system? [Pause.]

(5 minutes) On a piece of paper write down the first words that come to mind. These words do not need to 'make sense'.

(10 minutes) Think about who fed you and how. Were you fed by many different people? (You may have had one caregiver or many more.) Were you bottle fed with formula? Or breast fed?

Repeat the breath cycle three times.

Now take me to when you were a child. How old are you here?

Take me to when you ate food. This may be breakfast, lunch or dinner, or your favourite snack. Where are you? What are the sights and sounds? What do you smell? [Pause.]

Notice how you feel in your body. [Pause.]

Using a different sheet of paper, write the first words that come to mind.

Repeat the breath cycle three times.

Now imagine you're an adolescent. Where do you get your food? Do you eat dinner with your family, friends or on your own? What do you eat? Who makes this for you?

Repeat the breath cycle three times.

Now imagine you're an adult. What do you have for dinner? Do you cook? Does someone cook for you?

Repeat the breath cycle three times.

Now you are your present self, in the here and now. What do you tend to eat for lunch, dinner or breakfast? Select the first meal that comes to mind. What feelings come for you? What happens in your body? Take a moment to breathe. [Pause.]

(5 minutes) On your third separate sheet of paper, write down any words that come to mind.

(10 minutes) Repeat the breath cycle three times.

Imagine now your older self. [Please note: this may be an adult, older adult, etc. – adapt for your client.]

What do you imagine eating will look like for you in the future? Will you eat different food or eat similarly to how you do now?

What comes to mind? Notice your body. Can you easily imagine your older self, or is this more challenging?

(5 minutes) Using your fourth sheet of paper, write down words that come to mind.

Reflections and questions for the client (5 minutes)

- Look at the sheets of paper and the words you have written. Consider where the food you imagined comes from. Is this culturally connected to where you are from, your family, the society you grew up in? If so, how?
- How is each developmental stage different?
- Consider the similarities and what thoughts and feelings came up throughout. What themes arose?
- Did anything surprise you? If so, what?

Session 2 (30 minutes)

Take a few moments to look at the words laid out in front of you. For the next 20 minutes, use the art materials on one sheet of paper, or make one clay sculpture to explore what came up for you.

[When the 20 minutes has come to an end, invite your client to spend the next 10 minutes reflecting on the process.]

CHAPTER 6

Exploring Culture and Identity through Safety and Recognising What Is of Value to You

Therapeutic safety

Kristina Stamatiou and Natasha D'Aguiar

This activity uses a collaborative approach to exploring intersectionality in the client's safe relationships.

CREATING SAFETY (35 MINUTES)

Aim: To understand safety from the client's lived experience to find a way to meet their needs and actively find ways to create safety for them.

What you will need: Two sheets of paper, poster paints and a pen.

For the client (15 minutes): Think of someone who supports you, who comforts you, who makes you feel safe, who listens to you, who responds to your distress in useful ways. How do they respond to you? What do they say? How do they respond to you with their body? What is it about them that makes you feel better?

Is there anything about your relationship in terms of intersectionality or identity that helps you feel safe with them? Explore whether you have any shared intersections.

Split one sheet of paper in two by folding it in half. In the first column write the heading 'My person of safety'. Write the qualities down, including shared intersections or 'social graces' (see Chapter 1), that help in making this person safe for you. In the second column write the heading 'Therapeutic safety: what safety could look like from me [your therapist]'. What can I [the therapist] do that your safe person does? How can these qualities translate in therapy? Perhaps they can't, perhaps there are some differences – for example you are from the LGBTQIA+ community, as is your safe person, and the therapist is not. How can you bridge this gap? Perhaps you can't. Name this in the session. Can I [the therapist] work towards showing you those qualities?

Spontaneous artmaking using paints, for the client (10 minutes): Following on from the conversation about meeting your needs, including intersectionality and how your intersections differ or are similar, create art on the other sheet of paper using poster paints.

Reflections and questions for the therapist and client (10 minutes)

- How did this process feel for you?
- How did it feel to talk about this in the session?
- Look at the client's artwork. Does it reflect the conversation you had? Explore the painting's qualities with your client and if they can connect it to the conversation. It may or may not connect, and this is okay.

Emotional Emancipation Circles

Dr Sona Barbosa, clinical psychologist

I am African. I am an African woman. I am an African woman therapist. I am being the best version of myself.

It was within this frame of mind that I decided to apply to the Diploma in Black Psychology and African Centred Therapy. I hoped this course would offer me knowledge, focus and intention. I hoped it would provide me with tools which would enable me to better deal with current personal and professional challenges – such as being a Black practitioner in a white/Western-dominated world. I hoped.

What I got was so much more! I came in as an African woman. I was deconstructed and reconstructed as an extraordinary Black African woman practitioner. As the course progressed, the deconstruction and construction followed, and each session would bring new questions, discoveries, validations, identification. So many things made sense, so many emotions entangled, hope, joy, anger, frustration; alongside was the visible change on my therapeutic practice as well as on my personal life.

I have never been not proud to be a Black African woman, but I feel I never really grasped the limitless feeling of being proud to be one until recent years.

I remember the first day of the course. The excitement and the nervousness. And then the joy of seeing a room full of Black faces. The sense of relief and of belonging was overwhelming. It took me back to my first day of university, back in Portugal 28 years ago. The only Black person on the Clinical Psychology course in my year. The sense of displacement was real. This sense accompanied me throughout the course – the need to merge and understand who I felt I was and believed with what I was being taught was always in the back of my mind.

As Black African therapists I believe we have a responsibility to own the values and principles of the traditional healing practices and incorporate them into our personal and professional day-to-day lives.

I continue my journey towards my authentic African therapist self. I continue to integrate my learnings, not as theoretical concepts, but as my lived experiences. This will automatically be reflected in my therapeutic practice and, hopefully, benefit my clients. Within this context I would like to briefly share with you one of the tools I use when working with Afro-Caribbean communities.

Emotional Emancipation Circles (EECs)

> In the words of Dr Erica Mapule McInnis, 'The Emotional Emancipation Circles (EECs) were developed by ABPsi (Association of Black Psychologists) leaders in association with the Community Healing Network. They're becoming a global movement of safe spaces where black people work together on self-healing and emotional emancipation. Initially, they started as a response to help the community heal emotionally from human-made disasters such as unjust deaths of black people when interacting with law enforcement services and the uprisings which were often a way of the community expressing its hurt. Now, rather than waiting for problems to occur – and we know they inevitably will – the circles work on developing resilience skills pre-emptively.'
>
> What do they consist of? 'People telling stories, dancing, singing, practising African rituals. We practise mindfulness/resilience tools and share coping and wellness strategies, as well as learn more about how historical and social forces affect our relationships and emotions. It's critical that people feel safe in these circles, and also that they feel completely comfortable with saying what they want to say in front of other members. They are therefore black-only spaces.'[1]

EECs are evidence-informed, psychologically sound and culturally grounded self-help support groups designed to help people of African ancestry work together to overcome, heal from and overturn the root causes of the devaluing of Black Lives.

EECs are eight structured sessions of culturally centred peer support which provide an opportunity for participants to build self-worth, to connect and support each other by sharing stories and learn wellness skills. Participants also have an opportunity to train as EEC facilitators where they can lead their own sessions in the community.

---

1 www.bps.org.uk/psychologist/be-best-version-yourself-thats-what-african-psychology-does-me

EECs are designed to be led by laypeople. They are not intended to be – nor should they be treated as – a substitute for professional counselling, advice or therapy. Participants are urged to seek the help of qualified mental health professionals, if and when necessary. This unique approach demonstrates that there are alternatives to current therapeutic support systems which can improve access and outcomes to Black communities.

The EEC groups follow seven keys, which are affirmations designed to free group members from the psychological and emotional effects of centuries of racism. They are used within the groups to consciously remind the group circle of what they should understand and seek out, and how they can free themselves:

- Key 1: Truth, awareness – African spiritual origins
- Key 2: Justice, defiance – historical events
- Key 3: Balance, self-reflection – African cultural origins
- Key 4: Harmony, accountability – human development and learning character
- Key 5: Propriety, restoration – ethics and methods
- Key 6: Reciprocity, connection – the collective
- Key 7: Order, model and serve – spirit and spirituality.

THE ELEMENTS OF EVERY EEC (1 HOUR 30 MINUTES, GROUP ACTIVITY)

Setting the stage

- **Outreach:** In this context this means reaching those who are most impacted. Those from racial trauma, gendered oppression, intergenerational, ensuring the people entering this space are from these backgrounds. Outreach in EECs is the act of lovingly and intentionally inviting people into a collective healing space through trust, relationship and cultural resonance. This is so emotional emancipation can be shared, not imposed.

- **Facilitation preparation:** In this context this means for the facilitator to get ready to hold a scared trauma-informed healing space. This can be done by the facilitator grounding themselves, understanding the model and setting clear boundaries for the group where emotional emancipation can safely take place.

- Prepare the EEC space.
- Greet the attendees.

The opening (10 minutes)

- Background music, chosen by the facilitators, to remain the same each week.
- **Call to order:** Use the chosen song as mindfulness meditation for centring and focusing (2 minutes).
- Official welcome or introductions (in the first and second sessions, provide background information about what the EEC is and why people participate in it).
- Create and review the EEC shared agreements.

The activity (60 minutes)

- Share a toolkit topic, information and/or skill.
- Focus on an EEC key.
- Relate the key to an activity/information/sharing.
- Relate the key to the resilience toolkit information or skill. The 'key' is what brings the group together, following one of the seven keys listed. If what brings the group together is Key 1: Truth, awareness – African spiritual origins, then the toolkit information would be Information: Knowledge of African spiritual traditions and historical truths that counter internalised oppression; The Skill: Awareness, being able to name lived experiences, emotions and inherited narratives.

The closing (20–25 minutes)

- **Take away sharing or bring a tip exercise:** Take away sharing in this instance means what the participant has personally learned from this group, that they have an option or choice to share it within the circle and leave a practical tip exercise with the circle which can strengthen emotional and psychological resilience.
- Closing recitation.
- Closing song.
- Invitation to return next time and 'Each one, bring one'.

Evaluation

Attendees complete an EEC evaluation form. Here is an example of an EEC:

Key 6: Reciprocity, connection: Our African cultural imperative, connecting the collective
'From the story of "me" to the story of "we": random acts of kindness'
We create the world we desire through actions.

Doing for others heals the soul, soothes pain, lifts depression and reduces isolation. Ask yourself the following questions:

- What have I done for someone lately?
- What have I done for someone I didn't know – and they didn't know I had done it?
- Can you remember a time that something was done for you? What did it feel like?
- Share ideas of what people in the group could do. Why is this important?

We have to create the world we want to live in, despite the wrongs that are swirling around us.

Resilience tool: Grounding.

Special objects and items

Kristina Stamatiou and Natasha D'Aguiar

Objects and items are part of our everyday life. We usually wake up with the help of an object, an alarm clock or our phone (objects), we brush our teeth with a toothbrush (object), we wear our favourite perfume (object), put on our clothes and wear some jewellery (objects/items). By the time we leave home for the day, we have made contact with multiple objects. Some objects we may not think about much and others hold deeper, spiritual, religious or symbolic meaning.

YOUR SPECIAL OBJECTS AND ITEMS (50 MINUTES X TWO SESSIONS)

Aim: To deepen self-awareness and emotional connection through sensory exploration of meaningful objects. By engaging touch, memory and creative expression, participants reflect on personal attachments, inherited items and embodied responses. The process encourages mindfulness, grounding and storytelling, supporting insight into how objects carry personal and relational significance and how they contribute to one's sense of identity, safety and continuity across experiences.

What you will need: Clay, Play-Doh or carving material such as wood, ModRoc, rock and resin.

Session 1, Part 1 (20 minutes)

For the client: Close your eyes (if you feel safe to do so), breathe in for four and exhale for five. Repeat this process four times. Keeping your eyes closed, notice how the fabric of your clothes feels against your skin and body – does it feel soft, itchy or tight? Heavy or light?

With your eyes closed, think of an object or item you carry with you every day. How does this feel against your skin? Do you hold this or place it in a bag? Now think of an object or item that remains in your home, something you do not take out. Does it have its own spot or space within the home? How often do you see or notice it? Can you touch it? If not, why?

Pause for a minute and then repeat the breathing exercise: breathe in for four and out for five. Repeat this process five times.

Has anyone ever passed down an object or item to you? Who passed it down to you? Does it have a story?

Session 1, Part 2 (20 minutes)

For the client: Keeping in mind the objects or items you have just thought about, we would ask you to choose one of them to create a version of it using clay, Play-Doh or other carving material. You could create a replica of it if you wish, or you can create a symbolic object or item using the clay, Play-Doh or carving material to represent it.

Reflections and questions for the client (10 minutes)

- How did it feel to think about these different objects?
- Is there an object or item you believe you cannot be without? If so, which object or item?
- Is there an object or item you feel emotionally connected to? If so, which object or item?
- Has someone passed down an object to you? What is this? Who passed it down to you? What does it mean to you?
- What was it like to create your object based on the real one?
- What did the material feel like against your skin? Was it cold? Was it warm?

After this session has finished, please ask the client to bring with them to their next session their special object or item. If they cannot move it, could they possibly pick another smaller (and lighter) special object or item instead?

Session 2 (50 minutes)

For the client: You should have with you a special object you have brought into the session. Please hold it in your hands. Think about how it feels to be holding it. Notice anything that happens to your body as you are holding it (15 minutes).

Reflections and questions for the client (20 minutes)

- How did it feel to bring your special object to today's session?
- What was it like travelling with this object?
- How did it feel to hold this object in your hands?
- Did/does your body respond to this object? If so, in what way?
- Does anything happen to your body when you hold this object?
- Where in the body do you notice a response? Can you place your hand over this part of your body?
- How does it feel to place your hand over this part of your body? Does anything happen to your body?
- Does the object hold any special memories for you? If so, what are these?
- If you feel able, please share a memory you have based on this object or item.

Ending (15 minutes)

For the client: Please hold your object close to your chest, close your eyes and imagine becoming one with it. Visualise this object becoming part of you, forever keeping it safe within.

Spaces and places

Kristina Stamatiou and Natasha D'Aguiar

Spaces and places have shared an intimate relationship with people. Spaces and places can belong to one person or a whole community. Spaces and places form part of our identity and culture. We have domestic, working, spiritual, community, religious spaces and places, and more. Within these, further spaces and places can be found – for example domestic spaces and places may have wardrobes or kitchen drawers, religious spaces and places may have further worshipping spaces and private spaces, etc.... Every space and place we encounter holds a specific memory, dream or wish.

A GUIDE THROUGH SPACES (50 MINUTES)

Aim: To use creative exploration to examine the relationship between spaces, places and personal meaning, highlighting how environments hold memories, dreams and aspects of identity.

What you will need: Nothing, just your voice and your imagination.

Part 1 (20 minutes)

For the client: You can close your eyes or keep them open for this activity. Please visualise your domestic space. Imagine you are about to open your front door...you are now inside. Within your domestic space, please walk to your kitchen. Once you have reached your kitchen, please open up a cupboard of your choice. Have a look inside your cupboard – what do you see? Try to remember an item within your cupboard that you found. You are now going to walk to your bedroom. Visualise standing within your bedroom. Look around your bedroom – do you share your space with anyone else? Is there a window in your bedroom? If yes, look outside the window, look into the distance as much as you can before you can no longer see further. Is there anything you notice in the space ahead?

Part 2 (20 minutes)

For the client: For this part of the session, please take the therapist on a guided journey with you. Please imagine a different space – this could be a different space within the home or a spiritual place, for example. Please close your eyes and imagine yourself within that space...take your time. Notice any memories that come up for you or any dreams you may have had within these spaces and places...

Finally, open your eyes and look around the space you are currently in. Notice two things within the space and say what you notice aloud.

Reflections and questions for the client (10 minutes)

- What was it like moving through your chosen space?
- What was it like to travel through your chosen space with someone new?
- What does it feel like when you are in your chosen space?
- How does your body respond to your chosen space?
- Does anyone else share this space with you? If so, who?
- If you share this space with someone else, how does that feel?
- Would you like to share this space with anyone else? If so, who would this be?
- Are there any specific memories associated with your space? If so, what memories?

Identity: Looking within

Fazila Virmani (she/her), art psychotherapist

For me, identity has always been about exploring who I am in the world – both on a cultural level and within the intersected social structures of society, where navigating challenges can often be complex. I've found that creating portraits and figures provides a profound way to reflect inwardly as I work through questions of belonging – not just in society, but at various stages of my life. This process has been deeply inspired by my muse, Frida Kahlo, whose extraordinary self-portraits capture poignant moments of her life journey.

As an art psychotherapist, finding my place within various organisations has not been an easy path. Larger dynamics at play have shaped this experience, and through creating art, I've been able to visually place myself within those scenarios. This allows me to step back, observe from a different perspective, and rewrite the narrative.

This practice has not only helped me identify cracks and challenges within the structures I've worked in, but has also given me an insight into my own feelings. It has empowered me to step away from spaces that hinder my growth and to seek environments that foster it. I invite you, as therapists and practitioners, to draw inspiration from this process and use it in your sessions with clients – or even for yourself, as a means of self-reflection.

This activity focuses on the self-portrait, drawing attention to your face and how you look, what is portrayed visually through this part of your body. This explores a range of identities, but is not limited to race, gender, religion, ability and disability. What do you want to claim back in terms of your identity? What stereotypes are you wanting to dismantle? You then create a portrait claiming this back using collage as a medium. Collaging can provide a soothing, meditative experience, while also enabling clients to reimagine their circumstances and perspectives.

This activity can be used with all age groups. Younger children or adults may require additional support and guidance, but the process is adaptable and can be extended over several sessions. You and your client can collaborate to define the activity's aims, and as a therapist, you can create a safe and reflective space for processing and discussion at the end.

IMAGINARY MIRROR (50 MINUTES)

Aim: To use collage to create an image of your face. To empower the client (or yourself, the therapist) by creating a new visual narrative alongside their (or your) current one. To explore the stereotypes projected onto you and the biases connected to your outward appearance.

What you will need: Collage materials such as magazines or newspapers (or an electronic device and internet access if you prefer to do this virtually), scissors, A3 sheet of paper, glue.

Select about 10 images that you would like to use for your portrait (15 minutes).

Draw an outline of your face. This doesn't have to be perfect, a rough outline is good enough (5 minutes).

Arrange the images on the page and stick the images to the paper (20 minutes). Experiment with repetition through cutting and pasting in collage work, as the process itself can feel cathartic.

Reflections and questions for the client (10 minutes)

- Does your collage look similar or different to your real face? If so, how?
- How does it feel to look at your collage? What feelings come up for you?
- How did it feel to find the images you needed?
- What stereotypes came to mind, if any?

CHAPTER 7

Exploring Culture and Identity through Reflection

Motherhood through a cultural lens

Karen Raingold, art therapist

In my work as an art therapist specialising in the area of children and families, I have worked with parents and caregivers in a range of formats and settings, including therapy groups in community centres, parent consultations in schools and dyadic therapy sessions. While working with fathers is essential and valuable, and important to my practice, I wish here to explore working with mothers and 'motherhood' in particular.

Since becoming a mother myself, I have become personally aware of the unique physical, emotional and social demands of this role. From expectations and social discourse around fertility, pregnancy, pregnancy loss and child birth before we even have children (for non-adoptive mothers) to breastfeeding, sleep, boundaries and working/childcare schedules, there is huge pressure and overwhelming advice centred on mothers. The tone of this discourse is intersected by the culture/s from which mothers originate, as well as the one/s in which they are mothering, and the associations of gender that exist in these cultures.

It is important to take these into consideration when working with children and mothers, as they have a significant impact on their parenting, and therefore their children's attachments and internal working models. Here I want to encourage therapists to explore issues of culture, gender and inherited parenting approaches with mothers as a means of helping them to gain insight into their experiences of being mothered and of mothering.

To give myself as an example, although not practising, I am technically a 'Jewish mother' living in the UK. What this means socially and personally is complex. The 'Jewish mother' is a well-documented stereotype known for being anxious, sacrificing, demanding, manipulative and devoted. Today, it tends to carry largely negative associations, but actually originated from the historical notion of the 'Yiddishe Mama', which was a sentimentalised figure: a homemaker, known for her strength, creativity and moral force in the face of hardship and persecution (Sorkin 2023). It seems that as many of these struggles lessened for Jewish people, at least in the USA, these protective, anxious instincts became framed as neurotic and interfering and reflected negative attitudes to strong, outspoken women.

Another consideration in the mental health of contemporary Jewish mothers and their children is intergenerational trauma. According to research, descendants of people who survived the Holocaust have different stress hormone profiles than their peers (Rodriguez 2015). Other factors also affect the children and descendants of survivors, such as attachment being impacted by parents exhibiting frightening or frightened responses to stress and parents modelling patterns of feeling, thinking and behaving that originate as a result of trauma (e.g., distrust of others, pessimism and low self-esteem).

Being a middle-class mother in the UK, I am also exposed to the 'cult of the perfect mother', an impossible ideal that strives for breastfeeding, co-sleeping and staying at home on the one hand, and having a career and children who sleep, eat and 'behave' well on the other. These ideals are perpetuated largely through social media and are fuelled by modern research into the impact of parenting on children's social development. The result is that mothers often feel overburdened, anxious and guilty about their mothering, which is likely to have negative consequences for children in turn.

What greater forces may be behind this? Does it serve to distract mothers from other more material realities, that they are underpaid, overworked and undervalued? Constant searching for solutions to the needs of our children leads to big business for products for sleep, birthing, feeding, etc. These polarised ideals create identity confusion for mothers when perhaps it is healthiest to strive to be a 'good enough mother', one who recognises that their flaws are inevitable, and models to their children the importance of self-care, presence and making and repairing mistakes.

How does all this impact me and my mothering? Being able to explore and understand these influences and sociocultural factors is helpful for me in a number of ways. I can understand, from a biological and social perspective, the roots of my anxiety and perfectionism as a parent. With this I can enlist tools that will help me break free of negative cycles – such as limiting social media exposure, employing mindfulness and talking openly with friends and family. I can celebrate the strengths of my motherhood lineage, that is, the 'Yiddishe Mama', and recognise how and why society has skewed this. I can recognise that there are inherited elements of myself, my mothering and my children over which I have no agency, and I can work to accept and nurture rather than change these.

I recommend delivering this activity in three sessions, one for each element presented. Explain to the client that the purpose of the activity is to explore how they were mothered and the factors that influence how they mother, in order to identify what might be impacting their parenting style, attachments, responses and triggers.

EXPLORING MOTHERHOOD (50 MINUTES FOR EACH SESSION)

Aim: To create a starting point for supporting the client to think about two converging areas of their motherhood experience – the sociocultural factors present in how they themselves were mothered and those present currently for them as mothers. To look to the future and to explore what the client would like to pass on to their children.

What you will need: A medium- to large-sized box, collage materials, including magazines, scissors and glue, paper and a range of drawing materials, such as pencils, pastels, paints and inks, and sculpting materials, such as clay.

Session 1 (50 minutes)

Artmaking (30 minutes): Present the box and explain that it represents them as a mother. The outside of the box is for them to explore how they were mothered, visually, using the materials provided. (It is important to note that 'mother' in this context can refer to any maternal or caring figures in the client's childhood, including grandmothers, aunts, family friends, foster carers, etc.)

Reflections (15 minutes)

You may want to use the following questions as prompts for this or as prompts to begin a conversation about this before embarking on the activity:

- What comes to mind when you think of your 'mother'?
- How would you describe the style of parenting you received?
- What culture surrounded your mother when you were a child? How did that culture view the role of mother and women in general?
- Who else had a maternal influence on you, and how?

Ending (5 minutes): Before you finish for today, have a look at what you have made before we continue the activity next time. Reflect on if there were any surprises or if there is anything you would like to change. Notice what comes to mind as you look at what you've created; note this in your mind.

Session 2 (50 minutes)

Artmaking (30 minutes): The inside of the box is for the client to explore the influences on their own mothering.

Reflections (15 minutes): Here are some prompts for this element of the activity or conversation:

- Where did you learn to be a mother?
- What represents the ideal mother to you?

- What is going well for you as a mother and what is challenging?
- What representations of motherhood do you notice around you, and how do these make you feel?

Ending (5 minutes): Take a few moments to look at what you have created on the outside of the box, noticing what comes up for you. Acknowledge these thoughts before ending this part of the activity.

Session 3 (50 minutes)

Artmaking (30 minutes): Finally, the client can use the drawing, collage materials or clay to create messages, images or objects that represent what they would like to pass on to their child/ren to go inside the box. Clarify that this is not actually to be given to their child/ren, unless they wish to.

Reflections (10 minutes): Here are some prompts for this element of the activity or conversation:

- What do you wish your mother had told you about becoming a parent?
- What do you want your child/ren to know about you?
- What do you want your child/ren to know about life?
- What strengths do you want your child/ren to keep with them in life?
- How do you want your children to understand about their culture?

Ending (10 minutes): Look at the inside of the box and the box as a whole. Reflect on how this appears to you. Consider how it represents mothering, and whether that feels different from the way the box looks. Notice your thoughts and feelings.

Gifts and spirituality

Kristina Stamatiou and Natasha D'Aguiar

We are sent gifts of strength and also challenges from previous generations that we pass on to our children and our children's children – some of which are welcomed, some not so much. It can be tricky to find our strengths, and knowing where they come from can bring us connection to our beginnings and grounding for our future.

Perhaps some strengths have been gifted by ghosts of the past, those we didn't have a chance to meet or parents we didn't know. This activity allows the client to connect to their gifts. Whether the bestower is known or unknown, they can search for their energy and reconnect to their roots.

GIFTED STRENGTHS (45 MINUTES)

Aim: For the client to find the strengths that have been gifted to them from previous family generations.

What you will need: Ready-made cardboard boxes (at least five), a sheet of A4 paper and pen, paints, oil/soft pastels or colouring pencils.

Guided visualisation (10 minutes)

Read out the following to the client:

Softly allow your eyes to come to a close.

Take a breath in through your nose for 4 seconds and out through your mouth for 4 seconds. Repeat two times.

Allow yourself to imagine travelling through an environment – you can walk, cycle, drive, roller skate, anything you wish. Your surroundings can be somewhere that feels right for you – a beach, a park, a city...travel through acknowledging what's around you. [Pause.]

You follow a path and travel further and further. You see a box in the distance. [Pause.]

You notice the size, colour and texture. You travel closer towards it. As you move closer towards it you realise there is a name on the box. [Pause.]

The name is your name. You stop and open it. Inside you find words written to you from family members describing strengths they have passed down to you. You read the words. [Pause for 5 seconds.]

What does it say?

Artmaking (25 minutes): Please ask the client to list their gifts on a sheet of paper. Now they can decorate each cardboard box to represent each gift. This doesn't have to be literal; it can be abstract.

Reflections and questions for the client (10 minutes)

- Who are your gifts from and what are they?
- Who would you want to pass your gifts down to?

Family photos collage

Kristina Stamatiou and Natasha D'Aguiar

In this activity the client creates a collage that explores intersectionality within their family history, bringing this to modern-day images they are surrounded by. Please ask the client to bring together a selection of family photos (photocopies, not originals) and images of people they 'consume' on a daily basis. These may be people they follow on social media, see in newspapers or magazines, or from shows they watch.

MY FAMILY IN PICTURES (35 MINUTES)

Aim: To explore the client's intersecting identities by connecting family history with present-day influences through creative collage-making and family pictures.

What you will need: Access to a photocopier or printer, newspapers and magazines, scissors, glue and a sheet of A3 paper.

For the client (15 minutes): Find images of people from the same race/heritage/ethnicity as you and your family members. (You may want to do this before the session and bring the images with you.)

Now select headlines or words that are associated with your race/heritage/ethnicity in the media. (You may want to do this before the session and bring these with you.)

Cut out the images of your family members and of people in the media, then arrange them on the paper in a way that feels right for you. When you are happy with the arrangement, paste them on to the paper.

Now add the headlines onto the paper (10 minutes).

Reflections and questions for the client (10 minutes)

- How are people from your racial/ethnic background depicted in the press, social media and advertising, and how does this differ from your own family members?
- Do you see people of your race depicted in the media? Are they easy to find or difficult?
- How did this process feel?
- What emotions came up for you when viewing your images? Was it a surprise to see your race/ethnicity depicted in a certain way?
- Did this differ from how your family members present themselves?

Transforming inner scripts

Kristina Stamatiou and Natasha D'Aguiar

Often our thoughts and opinions about ourselves are derived from others, such as friends, family, social media, community and cultural influences. We begin to adopt and claim these beliefs and opinions as our own, and this, in turn, helps to develop a sense of self. These views become so deep-rooted that we internalise them, which shapes our worldviews, perceptions and behaviour.

Here, with the client, we are going to creatively explore some of the internalised inner scripts we have received from childhood up until now.

TRANSFORMING NEGATIVITY (50 MINUTES)

Aim: To enable the client to examine and creatively engage with internalised messages formed through relationships and social influences, fostering greater insight into their identity, worldview and behavioural patterns.

What you will need: Two sheets of paper, childhood photos (if accessible) and pencils or felt tip pens.

Step 1 (20 minutes)

If the client has access to photos of themselves when they were a child, ask them to choose one to bring to the session. If not, ask the client to draw themselves in the centre of a plain piece of paper or inside the photo frame we have created for them to use, leaving space around or outside the photo frame for writing.

If the client has picked one childhood photo of themselves, ask them to tape this in the centre of a plain piece of white paper or inside the photo frame. Ask them to write the age they were and their name below the photo.

Once this has been done, please ask the client to think of any negative messages they were told about themselves as a child. This could have been from a family member, a friend, a teacher or from social media. Ask them to write these messages around their photo. The messages could be linked to their gender, religion, appearance, accent, education and so on.

Step 2 (20 minutes)

On a separate piece of paper, ask the client to write to their childhood selves. Ask them to notice what they would like to say to their childhood version of themselves, thinking about what they would have liked to have heard from their family, friends, teachers and social media, instead of the painful and negative messages they may have received.

Step 3 (10 minutes)

Reflect on this activity with your client. Ask them to read the negative messages and the positive messages they wished they had received.

Questions for the client

- How did this activity feel?
- How did it feel to remember certain negative messages you were told about yourself?
- Could you feel anything happen to your body when you were remembering the negative messages? If so, where?
- How did it feel to rewrite your narrative with positive messages to your younger self?
- How did it feel within your body, when you were reading the positive messages back to yourself?

Acknowledgements and Afterword

We want to extend our thanks to all the contributors to this book – for their intimate sharing and their wondrous contributions; without them, this book would not have been possible. We would like to thank all the clients who shared their journeys with us, and who have taught us more about being therapists than any course could have.

Kristina: I would also like to particularly thank Leo Louca for reminding me of the importance of play, vulnerability and seeing the world again for the first time through the eyes of a young child. My thanks also go to Coco, Sally Louca, George Louca, Andreas Louca, Panayiota Stamatiou, Andy Stamatiou, Salomi Georgiou, Christakis Stamatiou; my late grandfather Giorgios Tsiarta and late grandmother Georgia Stamatiou, for their storytelling, experience and knowledge around their own Cypriot identity, which provided strong foundations for me to continue my own identity journey and curiosity; to my friends Zannetta Pavlakos, Melanie Boxer, Stella Roussou and Andrianna Davda, Sophia Sophroniou, the Poets; and finally, to Natasha, my co-author, who has been a pillar of strength throughout the writing process, and who also provided a home for me within her art therapist profession and the world.

Natasha: A very special thank you to Kristina for being the power, strength and organisation behind our partnership. You remind me that there is no glass ceiling for our duo, and you encourage me to grow and learn always. Aim as high as you can imagine, then aim higher still. You give me the courage to say things aloud that I didn't think I could. This book has been the product of our many conversations where we put the world to rights, where we gave voice to the rollercoaster of emotions we have experienced in the therapeutic arena, but also the realisation that we bring uniqueness and important voices that must be heard. Thank you for not allowing me to get too distracted! Thank you Matt Tarr for your unwavering support, for believing in me and for loving me for who I am and who we grow to be, and for listening to my many rants. Thanks for continuously reminding me that I can do anything. Without you encouraging me and building my confidence I wouldn't have thought I could do this. Thanks to my parents and their continued sacrifices in giving me a foundation where I'm not afraid to fail. Thank you to my therapy friends who have supported this book in many ways, for our conversations and showing endless kindness to the world around us all. You are the glue that holds the NHS together. And for the children, young people and families I have worked with: you are the inspiration for this book and why we have created this, to push the boundaries of therapy and to encourage better outcomes for those with mental ill health. I also couldn't have written this book without Ten the whippet, for his company and for giving me welcomed and unwelcome breaks during this whole process. Lastly, thank you to the cockroach in Cyprus for reminding us that every creature has the power to shake things up.

References and Further Reading

Agarwal, P. (2021) *Sway: Unravelling Unconscious Bias*. London: Bloomsbury Sigma.

Bachelard, G. (1964) *The Poetics of Space*. Translated from French by M. Jolas. Boston: Beacon Press.

Belkin, M. and White, C. (2020) *Intersectionality and Relational Psychoanalysis: New Perspectives on Race, Gender, and Sexuality*. London: Routledge.

Birdsey, N. and Kustner, C. (2021) 'Reviewing the social GRACES: What do they add and limit in systemic thinking and practice?' *American Journal of Family Therapy 49*, 5, 429–442. https://doi.org/10.1080/01926187.2020.1830731

Burnham, J. (1992) 'Approach–method–technique: Making distinctions and creating connections.' *Human Systems* 3, 1, 3–27.

Burnham, J. (2012) 'Developments in Social GRRRAAACCEEESSS: Visible-Invisible and Voiced-Unvoiced.' In I.-B. Krause (ed.), *Culture and Reflexivity in Systemic Psychotherapy: Mutual Perspectives* (pp.139–160). London: Karnac Books.

Cacace, A. and Summers, S. J. (2024) 'Intergenerational trauma in phenomenological research – A systematic review.' *Journal of Loss and Trauma 30*, 8, 1134–1169. https://doi.org/10.1080/15325024.2025.2490917

Cambridge Dictionary (no date) 'Creativity.' Cambridge: Cambridge University Press. https://dictionary.cambridge.org/dictionary/english/creativity

Campbell, D. (2012) 'Can We Tolerate the Relationships that Race Compels?' In I.-B. Krause (ed.), *Culture and Reflexivity in Systemic Psychotherapy: Mutual Perspectives*. London: Karnac Books.

Campbell, J. (1991) *The Power of Myth*. New York: Anchor Books.

Carey, N. (2011) *The Epigenetics Revolution: How Modern Biology Is Rewriting Our Understanding of Genetics, Disease and Inheritance*. London: Icon Books.

Crenshaw, K. (1989) 'Demarginalizing the intersection of race and sex: A Black feminist critique of antidiscrimination doctrine, feminist theory and antiracist politics.' *University of Chicago Legal Forum 1989*, 8. https://chicagounbound.uchicago.edu/uclf/vol1989/iss1/8

Eastwood, C. (2021) 'White privilege and art therapy in the UK: are we doing the work?' *International Journal of Art Therapy 26*, 2, 75–83. doi: 10.1080/17454832.2020.1856159

Erikson, E. H. (1950/1995) *Childhood and Society*. London: Vintage.

Freud, S. (1915/1957) 'The Unconscious.' In J. Strachey (ed. and trans.), *The Standard Edition of the Complete Psychological Works of Sigmund Freud, Vol. 14* (pp.159–215). London: Hogarth Press.

Govoni, R. M. and Weatherhogg, A. P. (2007) 'The body as theatre of passions and conflicts: Affects, emotions, and defences.' *Body, Movement and Dance in Psychotherapy* 2, 2, 109–121. doi: 10.1080/17432970701374486.

GOV.UK (no date) 'Discrimination: Your rights | Types of discrimination ("protected characteristics").' www.gov.uk/discrimination-your-rights

Groys, B. (2022) *Philosophy of Care*. London: Verso.

Halacre, M. (2020) *Working with Disability Across the Counselling Professions.* Good Practice across the Counselling Professions 007. https://www.bacp.co.uk/media/25543/bacp-working-with-disability-gpacp-007-nov-25.pdf

Hanna, J. L. (1988) *Dance, Sex, and Gender: Signs of Identity, Dominance, Defiance, and Desire.* Chicago, IL: The University of Chicago Press.

Hare, J. (2024) *Autism Is Not a Disease: The Politics of Neurodiversity*. London: Verso Books.

Heath, L. and Bunn, S. (2023) 'Factors shaping gender incongruence and dysphoria, and impact on health services.' POSTbrief 53. London: UK Parliament. https://researchbriefings.files.parliament.uk/documents/POST-PB-0053/POST-PB-0053.pdf

Hogan, S. (ed.) (2019) *Gender and Difference in the Arts Therapies: Inscribed on the Body*. London: Routledge.

Joseph, S. (2019) *Authentic: How to Be Yourself and Why It Matters*. London: Piatkus.

Krause, I.-B. (2012) *Culture and Reflexivity in Systemic Psychotherapy: Mutual Perspectives.* London: Routledge.

Lindkvist, M. (1998) *Bring White Beads When You Call Upon the Healer*. New Orleans, LA: Rivendell House Ltd.

Linklater, R. (2014) *Decolonizing Trauma Work: Indigenous Stories and Strategies*. Halifax: Fernwood Publishing Co. Ltd.

MBRRACE-UK (2024) *Perinatal Mortality Surveillance: UK Perinatal Deaths of Babies Born in 2023*. Maternal, Newborn and Infant Clinical Outcome Review Programme. 11 July. www.hqip.org.uk/wp-content/uploads/2025/05/Ref.-581-MNI-CORP-Perinatal-Mortality-Surveillance-Report_FINAL-1.pdf

McKechnie, D.G.J., O'Nions, E., Bailey, J., Hobbs, L., Gillespie, F. and Petersen, I. (2023) 'Transgender identity in young people and adults recorded in UK primary care electronic patient records: retrospective, dynamic, cohort study.' *BMJ Medicine* 2, e000499. https://doi.org/10.1136/bmjmed-2023-000499

Menakem, R. (2021) *My Grandmother's Hands: Racialized Trauma and the Pathway to Mending Our Hearts and Bodies*. London: Penguin.

NHS England (2025) *Trauma-Informed and Harm-Aware Inpatient Care*. www.england.nhs.uk/long-read/trauma-informed-harm-aware-inpatient-care

Office for Health Improvements & Disparities (2022) 'Working definition of trauma-informed practice.' 2 November. www.gov.uk/government/publications/working-definition-of-trauma-informed-practice/working-definition-of-trauma-informed-practice

ONS (Office for National Statistics) (2022) *Religion, England and Wales: Census 2021*. London: ONS. www.ons.gov.uk/peoplepopulationandcommunity/culturalidentity/religion/bulletins/religionenglandandwales/census2021

Pearson, J., Smail, M. and Watts, P. (2013) *Dramatherapy with Myth and Fairytale: The Golden Stories of Sesame*. London: Jessica Kingsley Publishers.

Prosho, C. (2024) *NHS Adult Gender Services in the UK: Performance Report*. July. Southsea: TransLucent Community CIC. https://translucent.org.uk/wp-content/uploads/2024/09/TransLucent-NHS-Adult-Gender-Services-in-the-UK-Performance-Report-Public.pdf

Rankine, C. (2020) *Just Us: An American Conversation*. London: Allen Lane.

Rober, P. (2012) 'Foreword.' In Krause, I-B. (ed.) *Culture and Reflexivity in Systemic Psychotherapy: Mutual Perspectives*. London: Karnac Books,. pp.xv–xvii.

Rodriguez, T. (2015) 'Descendants of Holocaust survivors have altered stress hormones.' Scientific American, 1 March. www.scientificamerican.com/article/descendants-of-holocaust-survivors-have-altered-stress-hormones

Rogers, C. R. (1961) *On Becoming a Person: A Therapist's View of Psychotherapy*. Boston, MA: Houghton Mifflin.

Rose, J. (2021) *The Intellectual Life of the British Working Classes*. 3rd edn. New Haven, CT: Yale University Press.

Royal College of Psychiatrists (2024) 'Is autism being overdiagnosed?' Equity, Diversity and Inclusion Blog, 19 April. www.rcpsych.ac.uk/news-and-features/blogs/detail/equity-diversity-and-inclusion-blog/2024/04/19/is-autism-being-overdiagnosed

Royal College of Psychiatrists (2025) '7.5 million referrals on waiting lists doesn't include mental health patients, cautions RCPsych.' www.rcpsych.ac.uk/news-and-features/latest-news/detail/2025/01/06/7.5-million-referrals-on-waiting-lists-doesn-t-include-mental-health-patients--cautions-rcpsych

Rubin, R. (2023) *The Creative Act: A Way of Being*. Edinburgh: Canongate Books.

Schwartz, P. and Schwartz, M. (2011) *The Dance Claimed Me: A Biography of Pearl Primus*. New Haven, CT: Yale University Press.

Sorkin, C. (2023) 'Confronting the Jewish mother stereotype.' Jewish Women's Archive, 12 July. https://jwa.org/blog/risingvoices/confronting-jewish-mother-stereotype

Stevens, A. (1994) *Jung: A Very Short Introduction*. Oxford: Oxford University Press.

Tajfel, H. (2010) *Human Groups and Social Categories: Studies in Social Psychology*. Cambridge: Cambridge University Press.

Tajfel, H., Billig, M. G., Bundy, R. P. and Flament, C. (1971) 'Social categorization and intergroup behaviour.' *European Journal of Social Psychology 1*, 2, 149–178. https://doi.org/10.1002/ejsp.2420010202

Taylor, K.-Y. (2017) *How We Get Free: Black Feminism and the Combahee River Collective*. Chicago, IL: Haymarket Books.

Tempest, K. (2022) *On Connection*. London: Faber & Faber.

Turner, D. (2021) *Intersections of Privilege and Otherness in Counselling and Psychotherapy*. London: Routledge.

Tweedy, R. (2017) *The Political Self: Understanding the Social Context for Mental Illness*. London: Karnac.

van der Kolk, B. A. (2014) *The Body Keeps the Score: Brain, Mind, and Body in the Healing of Trauma*. New York: Viking.

WHO (World Health Organization) (2018) *Adverse Childhood Experiences International Questionnaire (ACE-IQ)*. www.who.int/publications/m/item/adverse-childhood-experiences-international-questionnaire-(ace-iq)

Wickenden, M. (2023) 'Disability and other identities – How do they intersect?' *Frontiers in Rehabilitation Sciences 4*, 1200386. https://doi.org/10.3389/fresc.2023.1200386

Winnicott, D. W. (1971) *Playing and Reality*. London: Tavistock Publications.

Women and Equalities Committee (2023) *Black Maternal Health: Third Report of Session 2022–23*. https://publications.parliament.uk/pa/cm5803/cmselect/cmwomeq/94/report.html

RAISING READERS

Books Build Bright Futures

Dear Reader,

We'd love your attention for one more page to tell you about the crisis in children's reading, and what we can all do.

Studies have shown that reading for fun is the **single biggest predictor of a child's future life chances** – more than family circumstance, parents' educational background or income. It improves academic results, mental health, wealth, communication skills, ambition and happiness.[1]

The number of children reading for fun is in rapid decline. Young people have a lot of competition for their time. In 2024, 1 in 10 children and young people in the UK aged 5 to 18 did not own a single book at home.[2]

Hachette works extensively with schools, libraries and literacy charities, but here are some ways we can all raise more readers:

- Reading to children for just 10 minutes a day makes a difference
- Don't give up if children aren't regular readers – there will be books for them!
- Visit bookshops and libraries to get recommendations
- Encourage them to listen to audiobooks
- Support school libraries
- Give books as gifts

There's a lot more information about how to encourage children to read on our website: **www.RaisingReaders.co.uk**

Thank you for reading.

hachette UK

1 OECD, '21st-Century Readers: Developing Literacy Skills in a Digital World', 2021, https://www.oecd.org/en/publications/21st-century-readers_a83d84cb-en.html

2 National Literacy Trust, 'Book Ownership in 2024', November 2024, https://literacytrust.org.uk/research-services/research-reports/book-ownership-in-2024